MASSAGE THERAPY

The Basics of the Best Massage Techniques in the World: Swedish, Deep Tissue, Trigger Point, Acupressure, Reflexology, and Percussion. Relieves Your Joint Pains and Relaxes Your Muscles.

By

Walter Bishop

© Copyright 2020 by Walter Bishop

All rights reserved.

This document is geared towards providing exact and reliable information with regard to the topic and issue covered. The publication is sold with the idea that the publisher is not required to render accounting, officially permitted, or otherwise qualified services. If advice is necessary, legal or professional, a practiced individual in the profession should be ordered.

From a Declaration of Principles which was accepted and approved equally by a Committee of the American Bar Association and a Committee of Publishers and Associations.

In no way is it legal to reproduce, duplicate, or transmit any part of this document in either electronic means or in printed format. Recording of this publication is strictly prohibited, and any storage of this document is not allowed unless with written permission from the publisher. All rights reserved.

The information provided herein is stated to be truthful and consistent, in that any liability, in terms of inattention or otherwise, by any usage or abuse of any policies, processes, or directions contained within is the solitary and utter responsibility of the recipient reader. Under no circumstances will any legal responsibility or blame be held against the publisher for any reparation, damages, or monetary loss due to the information herein, either directly or indirectly.

Respective authors own all copyrights not held by the publisher.

The information herein is offered for informational purposes solely and is universal as so. The presentation of the information is without a contract or any type of guarantee assurance.

The trademarks that are used are without any consent, and the publication of the trademark is without permission or backing by the trademark owner. All trademarks and brands within this book are for clarifying purposes only and are owned by the owners themselves, not affiliated with this document.

Table of Content

INTRODUCTION 1

What Is Massage Therapy? 4

History of Massage Therapy 7

The Fundamental Difference Between Physiotherapy and Massage Therapy 11

The Benefits of Massage Therapy on the Body 14

Massage Therapy – How It Works 19

Popular Types of Massage Therapy 21

Swedish Massage – For Relaxation and Wellbeing 23

    The Hallmarks of Swedish Massage and How Can It Benefit You 27

    Swedish Massage in a Massage Chair Recliner 29

    The Moves of Swedish Massage 32

Deep Tissue Massage 37

    Deep Tissue Massage - Muscle Tendon and Ligament Relief 37

    Deep Tissue Massage for Pain Relief 40

    Using Deep Tissue Massage Therapy to Reduce Musculo-Skeletal Pain 42

    Who Benefits from Deep Tissue Massage Therapy? 44

    Massage Chair Performs Deep Tissue Massage 47

    How Does Deep Tissue Massage Differ from a Standard Massage? 50

    The Health Benefits of Deep Tissue Massage 51

    How to Choose Between Swedish and Deep Tissue Massage Therapy 52

What Is Trigger Point Therapy?..55
    Trigger Point Therapy with Acupuncture Can Reduce Your Pain......59
    Trigger Point Therapy - Knot to Be Overlooked.................................60
Acupressure Massage Therapy Restore Balance and Harmony.................64
    Massage Chairs Incorporate Acupressure Massage Therapy................66
    Points, Sports, and Acupressure Massage..69
    Effectiveness of Acupressure..71
    Acupressure Therapy - Health in Your Hand and Feet.........................74
    Benefits of Receiving Acupressure Treatments......................................77
Reflexology...80
    What Is Reflexology?...80
    Reflexology - The Art of Foot Massage..82
    Reflexology Is Much More Than Just a Foot Massage.........................84
    Reflexology for the Feet..87
    Foot Reflexology Systems in Massage Chairs..90
    What Is the Difference Between Massage and Reflexology?................93
    Does Foot Reflexology Work?...94
    Modern Reflexology..96
    Hand Reflexology - A Healing Art..97
    Foot Reflexology..99
    Chinese Reflexology Therapy..100
    The Benefits of Hand Reflexology..102
    The Difference Between Foot and Hand Reflexology........................103

Percussion Massage Therapy 107

Massage Therapy – Preparing the Area 110

Are There Risks Involved in Massage Therapy? 112

Understand What to Expect During Massage Therapy..........................115

What Is the Best Type of Massage Therapy for Me? 118

When Should You Get Massage Therapy? 122

Mobile Massage Therapy..124

    Bodywork as a medical therapy 125

    Pregnancy bodywork 127

CONCLUSION 128

INTRODUCTION

Recently, massage therapy in the United States has developed exponentially. It has become more widely accepted by both physicians and the general public as a medical practice.

Massage is characterized as:... 'systematic manual or mechanical manipulation by movement such as rubbing, punching, pulling, slapping, and taping of soft tissues in the body, for therapeutic purposes such as promoting the blood and lymph circulation, muscle relaxation, pain relief, restoration of the metabolic equilibrium and other advantages, both physical and mental.'

The origins of massage can be traced back to ancient cultures, where many artifacts were found to support the belief that primitive people were using some type of oil and massaging their muscles.

Massage therapy was common throughout the years and was officially acknowledged by the first National Therapeutic Massage and Bodywork Certification in 1992.

Massage therapy provides many benefits without drugs for the human body. "Massage therapy has clearly proven to be very beneficial for me, particularly in areas of non-successful conventional medicine, including chronic arthritis, musculoskeletal syndrome and chronic headache".

Massage is a normal and instinctive way to relieve mild discomfort and pain, nerve stress and fatigue. Direct benefits include increased blood circulation, muscle tissue stretching, and scar tissue loosening. This leads to the indirect effects of lower blood pressure and general muscle relaxation.

The main benefits of massage therapy include increased nervous system, muscle system health, and circulatory system health. The stimulation of the muscle system and its circulation, nerve supply, and cell activity promotes muscle nutrition and growth.

Injured muscle tissue will have a quicker healing time and fewer complications when therapeutic therapy is administered because the development of scar tissue is stopped or disconnected.

Massage also prevents damage to a ligament or tendon by dispersing inflammation due to injury Because of the advantages that muscular system massage therapy offers, massage is an efficient means of improving muscle tone, muscle resistance and strength.

Massage can avoid, or at least delay muscle atrophy that results from inactivity. Massage also helps to ease muscle cramps or spasms or even to eliminate them. Depending on the type of treatment used, the nervous system can be stimulated or soothed. Massage activates skin and muscle nerve endings.

As quickly as acupuncture can activate the nerve, this can allow the nervous system to sedate and even alleviate insomnia. The consistency and amount of blood circulating through the circulatory system is influenced by the therapeutic massage.

Massage dilates blood vessels, boosting blood circulation". An increase in blood flow leads to the increased blood supply and the nutrients provided by muscles and other important bodies.

Through its long history, therapeutic massage has become a common and fairly safe relaxation process. Massage is actually virtually accessible in all fields including spas, health clubs, restaurants, hospitals, dental offices, and even airports.

For thousands of years, massage therapy has proven to be an effective method of treating many disorders and continues to be used for thousands of years to come.

This GUIDE explores the basics of massage therapy focusing on the major types and its benefits.

Let's get started!

CHAPTER 1

WHAT IS MASSAGE THERAPY?

Anyway, what is massage therapy? One thing we can say for sure, is that the profession has grown rapidly. You never learned about massage therapy a few decades ago. Yet awareness has grown tremendously since then. Even insurance companies know the benefits of a skilled massage therapist and recognize them.

The word massage therapy applies to health and healing procedures involving touch and movement. It is a discipline in which the therapist uses some manual methods and can be used for adjunctive therapy. Such strategies are used primarily in order to make a positive impact on the safety and well-being of the consumer.

The word massage is likely to come from the word "Massein," meaning "to knead" or "to press" in Arabic. Massage is probably man's oldest known form of physical medicine. It can be traced back to around 400BC throughout the early Chinese medical manuscripts. Hippocrates is considered to be in favor of massage.

And in the fifth century, he was born and also known as "the medicine guy." It was used and written about in Roman times, Julius Caesar's history recording was massed to help relieve neuralgia!

Thousands of years have passed after the massage therapy. The term massage was referred to in ancient writings from many cultures.

In the United States, massage therapy became popular for several health purposes in the mid-1800s. It included: ancient Greek old Rome China Japan

Indian subcontinent. Massage therapy fell out of favor around the 1930s and 1940s.

This was due to scientific and technological advancements in medical treatments. The interest in massage therapy was revived in the 1970s. Athletes used this form of therapy primarily at the time.

More than 80 styles of massage therapy are available. Most of the time, when people find a technique or two they prefer, they always hold to their therapist who uses this form of therapy. Then sometimes people find a certain massage therapist who makes them feel relaxed and who stays loyal to this specific massage therapist.

The first thing to happen is that the massage therapist should discuss the symptoms and needs. Then you are asked about your problem and circumstances.

There are a number of massages used to help: minimize stress and pain increase blood flow calming muscles and give a sense of health and relaxation. Massage therapy is really a hands-on treatment of soft tissues and body joints.

Although it significantly affects those muscles just below the skin, massage treatments may also help the deeper layers of muscle and perhaps also the organ itself. Soft tissue includes muscle tendons connected with fascia ligaments joint capsules.

Massage promotes blood circulation and helps to eliminate waste throughout the body by the lymph system (which runs parallel to the circulatory system).

Massage therapy is intended to prevent, develop, sustain, rehabilitate, or improve physical function, or alleviate pain. It is also a clinical option with an undeniable result in alleviating a variety of discomforts including stress, muscle overuse and many other chronic pain syndromes.

The massage therapist can force, stroke, rub to try and manipulate the muscles and other soft tissues, especially in the area of muscles and pressure points.

Pressing, and relieving of pain, relaxing, kneading stimulation and toning of the body. This is often done with different pressure and movement. The therapists use their palms, their thumbs, their shapes, their elbows and sometimes their feet.

In order to calm the soft tissues, help improves the blood and oxygen supply in the massaged areas, minimize stress, relieve muscles, decrease discomfort and provide a sense of well-being and relaxation.

Some of the famous massage styles are Swedish Deep Tissue Trigger Reflexology. You should only have the massage today with someone who uses the title of "massage."

This person has completed a diploma course and passed an examination at a recognized school. If you're looking for a qualified therapist, try someone whose occupation is a massage therapist (MT) or a licensed massage therapist (RMT).

Please be sure to consult your doctor before initiating a massage program if you experience certain circulatory conditions (such as phlebitis), infectious illnesses, certain forms of cancer, heart problems, certain skin conditions or any infected or inflamed tissue. A skilled massage therapist can also inform you if the massage is not shown.

CHAPTER 2

HISTORY OF MASSAGE THERAPY

Massage is one of the oldest art forms with the human body and often underestimates its benefits. Massage history comes from Asia, particularly China and India. Some ask exactly what massage therapy is because the term is commonly used in areas like spas and hospitals.

This blends human touch with muscle movement to create a calm state of mind. To learn, you need to learn their different definitions, practices and therapeutic effects, which practitioners have known throughout history.

The source of massage, in particular, medical care, is often traced to the Eastern Chinese medical practice of 2000 BC. However, many benefits may not all benefit from medical-massage.

The human touch element, for example, has little to do with how you learn and how personally the massage therapist is and how much energy it brings into the room. Kneading muscles and skin, using a warmer top-of-the-line massage table or the perfect combination of towels and lighting does not work if the guest is not relaxed.

The practitioner must also practice massage therapy in a way that will calm and provide their patients with positive energy. No matter what type of massage you do, patients usually see you help relax and alleviate the pain.

Methods of practice include: medical treatment, back pain therapy, chronic massage therapy, stress relief treatment, and other similar practices, such as aromatherapy (scented oil massage), Reiki (foot massage) and other types.

There is a great discussion about the efficacy of back pain treatment in the medical community. A US government health department Pub Med paper, for example, analyzed a group of patients with chronic back pain treatment and found that their condition was substantially supported and their back pain was less severe. Indeed, the Ontario College of Massage Therapists found that it was necessary to learn on back pain to learn massage therapy and to help these patients effectively.

Continuous education has shown that 92 percent of patients have increased performance, decreased discomfort, and reduced pain sharpness during massage therapy in this study.

Practices of healing or took place in the year 2000 BC, which continue today. Most medical massage therapists treat pain treatment, sports injuries or other chronic pain. Such therapists also gain certification and practice counseling in various schools and educational programs.

But British Columbia, Canada, is the longest program in the world, and it takes three years to learn massages. Although this seems like a long program, continuing massage training is an important part of every program.

Healers in Eastern cultures are often priests or spiritual leaders of their families who practice medicine. As Vancouver, Canada researcher Paul Ingram states, however, massage benefits are "temporary and incoherent" and can vary from patient to patient, from clinic to clinic for massage therapy, from therapist to therapist.

The current trends extend beyond massage history and use historical techniques with modern medicine to establish well-balanced practices between the two.

To practice massage, therapists today should be open to a wide variety of techniques, instruments, and purposes. While massage used to be a simple concept, the new combination of Western and Eastern history of massage therapy and modern techniques enabled diversity.

When we go back into history, we discover that since Christ's time, massage therapy has been around. Bodywork therapy in the United States first became known throughout many ancient civilizations in the mid-19th century.

Some massage treatments, such as Ayurvedic Abhyang massage, are thousands of years old in India and are given by one or two therapists. This unique body massage combines warm herbal oils with gentle kneading and pressures. The feet are sometimes used for the treatment, such as the Hawaiian Lomi massage technique.

Craniosacral therapy is commonly referred to as a unique type of massage therapy, often used in the wellbeing of an osteopathic practitioner. Craniosacral therapy is known to free tension from the spinal cord and optimize spinal fluid flow as a hand-held treatment involving light touch to help hydraulic forces within the natural cranial sacral system.

The technique of deep tissue is one of the most common types of massage therapy and is usually taught in most somatic programs. This particular modality of bodywork requires greater use of fingertips, knuckles, or elbow strain.

Reflexology is an energy-based massage therapy that is most commonly given to the feet' soils; however, it is also given to the hands, ears and body. Reflexology is a treatment that encourages stresses on the foot surfaces and claims that different feet pressure points suit parts of the body that can help relieve pain and stress in such areas.

Chinese medical massage therapy, also known as Tuina, is similar to acupressure and is applied at the sites of these body acupressures through kneading, pushing, and stretching techniques. Tuina's also based on energy healing is based on the philosophy that these points of acupressure are related to organ systems and parts of the body.

There are, of course, several other modes of massage therapy available today. You should check with your local certified massage therapist to find out which massage technique is best for you, who can explain the various techniques she uses in her practice.

As with most practitioners, massage therapists must comply with state education or license requirements before practicing the healing technique. Although many massage practitioners are present, it is important to note that there are no two massage practitioners alike.

In Swedes, deep tissue and sports massages certified, more specialized practitioners may offer additional services in acupressure, shiatsu, hot stone massage, neuromuscular therapy and myofascial release.

.

CHAPTER 3

THE FUNDAMENTAL DIFFERENCE BETWEEN PHYSIOTHERAPY AND MASSAGE THERAPY

Among the greater numbers of people, there is a very common misunderstanding about physiotherapy and massage therapy. It is not the same treatment and it is impossible to achieve all the advantages of both treatments.

Although both therapies can perform nearly the same tasks. The following post illuminates the fundamental difference between physiotherapy and massage therapy.

Massage and physiotherapy Massage and physiotherapy are both medical tools used by thousands of practitioners to improve one's health.

Physiotherapy is a well-known medical profession used by registered and licensed physiotherapists who treat their patients to remove various body injuries, pains and headaches, including therapy or therapeutic drug work.

Comparison Between Massage and Physiotherapy Several manual procedures were also used according to the patient's condition. Massage therapy, however, is nothing other than an alternative medicine consisting of organized body movements used for the stimulation of body muscles and ligaments.

Likewise, physiotherapists do create individualized and tailored programs for each patient so that movement and function can be restored to the body. Age, body weight, illnesses, and accidents all involve a very limited movement of the human body.

Several therapies are available to enhance a person's well-being, rehabilitation, manual interventions, and practical preparation. However, many physiotherapists specialize in the reintegration of pelvic floors, custom bracing, acupressure, acupuncture and myofascial discharge.

Physiotherapy Advantages

There are several physiotherapy advantages. This supports people with back pain, neck pain, shoulder injuries, arthritis, sclerosis, burn, sprains, fractures, and other injuries associated with regular work or exercise.

A physiotherapist also creates various retraining programs as well as restricted motion, avoids any loss of mobility, decreases body pain, and eliminates future disorders.

The advantages of massage therapy are nothing more than a procedure used by trained and licensed professionals. It involves different techniques for moving muscles, soft tissues, and other body aches.

Massage therapy techniques may include rub, knead, roll, shake, vibrate, vibrate, compress, and sometimes active and passive deformation within the normal anatomical range of motion.

Swedish massage, trigger massages, deep-tissue massage, and head massage performed by most massage therapists around the world are among the most common forms of massage therapy.

Such treatment will treat different types of disorders. It also helps you alleviate your muscle tightness, body aches, reduce pain and muscle spasms, boost your immunity, improve your blood pressure, enhance your blood flow, ease your discomfort, feel sorry during your pregnancy and improve your athletic performance.

Massage therapy can help you get back from intense workouts. It's also good to deal with anxiety, headache, and depression.

Last but not least, after complete medical examination, body assessment and diagnosis, and physical intervention, physiotherapy is particularly performed. Massage therapy, however, is nothing more than a common, practical approach used for exhaustion, work-life balance, relaxation, stress management, bodywear and feel good.

These procedures are used sometimes to improve soft tissue function, alleviate muscle pain, decrease stress and spasm, these medically and athletically.

It is commonly used for medicinal purposes. A trained and accredited health service provider can only encourage you to choose the appropriate treatment for your needs, be it physiotherapy or massage therapy.

Chapter 4

The Benefits of Massage Therapy on the Body

Massage therapy is an alternative medicine that has quickly gained popularity. The massage therapy field has grown not only in size but also in the availability of therapists, massage studios and massage clinics.

There is no doubt that most people would like a massage. Something people don't realize with the massage is that it doesn't only feel good and relax the body, mind, and spirit, but that it also strengthens the body, muscles and soft tissues.

Massage therapy is from the B.C. Age of history, Roman, Greek, Indian, Japanese, Chinese, Egyptian, and Mesopotamian civilizations. Massage is now throughout the world. Massage in China is considered a primary health care element and is taught in medical schools.

In the 1800s, massage therapy was introduced in the United States. However, its progress was slow and rocky in the American medical scene. Due to advances in technology in medicine, the massage declined throughout the early 1900s but regained its reputation in the early 60s and 70s when professional athletes started using massage therapy throughout their health routine.

The inexperienced characters that used massage therapy to advertise sexual services were extremely deterrent to massage therapy as alternative medicine and as a profession.

The purchase and sale of sex or sexual services in the USA and several other countries are illegal. Thus massage rooms offer sexual services after the purchase of a massage using the cover of massage treatment.

This kind of service, which damaged its reputation, became infamous for a time. With time, real massage therapists reclaimed their reputation as a holistic healing medicine slowly but surely.

Massages are now an immense industry, with thousands of schools, hospitals, and clinical facilities and licenses and qualifications in every Country. While there are still massage rooms, their existence remains largely in ghettos and seedy hoods.

Today when you talk about massage therapy, people do not think about sexual favors but instead about a soothing and enjoyable experience. Massage therapy has regained its reputation as an art of healing by body and muscle tissue manipulation.

The typical person would tell you that massage therapy always involves rubbing the whole body with soothing lotion or cream, which feels good. This massage interpretation, although correct in terms of the layman, does not explain what massage therapy is or how it affects the body.

The massage treatment team manipulates the body's soft tissues to boost performance, facilitate relaxation, reduce muscle spasms, pain and inflammation, reduce nervous tension, lower myofascial trigger points, improve mobility and joint flexibility.

Manual manipulation of soft tissue by pressure, stress, motion, and vibration is part of the massage process. Based on specific patient issues, the areas in which a massage therapist operates will be decided.

Techniques can depend on the type of massage be employed by the hands, fingers, elbows, knees, forearms or feet. The particular tissue is also determined to decide whether a muscle, tendon, ligament, skin, joints, connective tissue, lymph vessels or organ is concerned.

Several forms of massage techniques exist. Ayurvedic, deep tissue, sports massage, myofascial release, activating point therapy, reflexology, medical massage, Swedish massaging, stone massage, Thai massage, and shiatsu all form traditional massage techniques.

In addition to procedures, there are also several different strokes, such as effleurage, petrissage, tapotage, acceleration, trigger point care, neuro-muscular, manual lymph drainage, and manual traction, to be used by massage therapists.

Although massages are known as complementary and alternative medicines (CAM), they are becoming more and more a part of the medical world. The massage covers health clubs, health clinics, dentist offices, private offices, nursing homes, sports facilities and hospitals.

In tandem with many other medical professions such as chiropractor, acupuncture, physical therapy, personal training, and athletic trainers, massage therapy is hired.

Whatever the reason for a massage, it is a great treatment to relieve stress, pressure, headaches, neck pain, back pain, anxiety, and several other mental or physical problems. If you haven't had a massage yet, you've had one.

Most people have massages in their wellness schemes because they are not only good for the body, but also for the mind and spirit. As your mates for a therapist's suggestions close you!

There are several health benefits of massage therapy. This supports your intellectual, physical, and emotional well-being if you regularly consider doing so. It can be regarded as a good option for different drugs with harmful side effects.

The health benefits you receive are the same, whether it is a Swedish massage or a sports massage. This chapter explores some of the major advantages of massage therapy.

Firstly, the blood supply is boosted by massage therapy. When the massage is finished, the body muscles are relaxed, and blood supply to all parts of the body is increased.

Good blood flow means that all cells are supplied with oxygen, and other life-saving nutrients and waste materials are removed very effectively from the body. Enhanced nutrient supply to all parts of the body would improve health.

Massage is very effective in reducing stress. A quick massage can more easily free your mind from negative emotions. Since massage therapy relaxes close muscles, tension-related headaches are extremely effective.

Massage is also known for its pain relief quality. Massage is sometimes used in combination with other therapies, including physical therapy, hydrotherapy, etc.

It is also considered an important treatment for the control of pain in patients with muscle spasms, inflammation, and sciatica. Massage therapy can reduce lower back pain. The relief of pain is caused by the release of endorphins, primarily by endorphins, which are the natural painkillers of the body.

The treatment also increases one's immunity. The massage activates the lymphatic circulation, which is considered a mechanism of body defense. Massage therapy is also supposed to increase the amount of your WBC.

Massage has a calming and sedative effect on your central nervous system. A quick massage can either relax or activate the nervous system. The effects on the CNS depend directly on the current status, the form of treatment and the length of your nervous system. This plays well to relax a patient aggressively.

Massage therapy increases the range of motion of your joint and makes the body more flexible. It extends the connective tissues that support the muscles, increasing the flexibility of your body.

If you have cross-sectional massage strokes, you can prevent muscle fibers from attaching more. It guarantees the full range of motion and strength of your muscles.

CHAPTER 5

MASSAGE THERAPY – HOW IT WORKS

Massage therapy is a part of life: people who donate, give one to another, or seek professional services and almost everybody loves it. The therapy promises pain relief, headaches and other conditions, but how? Issues that help people to understand the field are what massage therapy is, what the advantages are and how it works.

Massage therapy is characterized as muscle and connective tissue manipulation to enhance body relaxation and function. This is basically how the therapy works. Provision or massage helps to calm the body by relieving muscle tension and improving mobility in many ways.

Therapists typically use one central treatment approach but also combine methods. The hybrid approach helps relieve more patient symptoms and illnesses because each technique has a different overall purpose to benefit a person.

Many forms focus on many different areas of the body for an individual's physical and mental health. Massage therapy has been shown to benefit patients in many ways through studies.

This promotes health by enhancing circulatory healing injuries that enable the immune system to combat disease, improve joint flexibility and reduce stress, thereby helping the therapy function. Medical experts attribute 80 to 90% of the disease to stress. Therapists practice and regularly learn new techniques to help their patients.

Most colleges offer a wide variety of qualifications and grades that prepare students for the rapidly growing field of medicine. Through this natural healing training, people can work in a range of jobs and professions.

Therapists will participate in physical therapy, athletic training and a wide variety of recreational activities. There are many paths to pursue and some include deep tissue, Russian, Swedish massage and shiatsu preparation.

Students learn these techniques and learn more to help patients achieve good overall health. Let's look in-depth at the above choices. The popular deep tissue massage is used to relieve the muscle and connective tissue from severe tension.

This works by reaching the muscles below the top muscle layer. It form of treatment is used in persons with persistent pain associated with persons doing many things, such as athletes or disabled persons.

A Russian massage uses a three-phase procedure. The first phase is slow and gentle, followed by a complicated, profound and rapid phase and finishes more slowly than in the first step. The popular Japanese shiatsu therapy includes thumb, finger, palm and stretching pressure.

Swedish massage is one of the oldest and has five stroking styles. Sliding, kneading, movement, friction, and vibration are all of these strokes. The approach allows patients to relieve pain, relax joints, and increases their mobility in osteoarthritis patients.

Massage therapy uses many different techniques to help people improve their general relaxation and well-being.

Chapter 6

Popular Types of Massage Therapy

More than 80 forms of massage therapy are available today. Massage therapies, including Swedish massages, deep tissue massages, sports massage acupressure, reflexology, and the chair massage, are some of those most popular in the massage industry.

For instance, Acupressure massage therapy is based on theories of Traditional Chinese Medicine (TCM) and not only is used for people but also as a form of canine and equine massage.

Use meridian therapy as a technique to depress key points on the body to relieve tension and challenges and to restore the body's energy flow (Chi) is thought to restore equilibrium and natural healing abilities in this particular type of massage.

Reflexology is another form of massage therapy, which is also rooted in oriental medicine. Specific feet sole areas (reflex zones) correspond with specific organ systems in the body.

It is assumed that these respective organ systems can be stimulated to recovery by applying pressure techniques to these reflex areas. This specific massage therapy is applied on the feet; reflexology is also provided to the hands, face and body.

In addition to Swedish massage techniques, a sports massage incorporates a variety of other touch therapies such as compression, cross-fiber therapy, hydrotherapy, and pressure points methods among others. Athlete also needs massages, such as sports massage treatments. Sports massage therapy is also offered to animals, including acupressure.

Deep tissue therapy is one of the basic bodywork therapies taught today in virtually all massage and healing schools. As the name implies, this is a deep muscle treatment that works to alleviate chronic pain and stress in the connective tissues and muscles.

Chair massage therapy, also known as a sitting massage, takes place at airports, business functions and in shopping malls. This bodywork is done while the customer sits upright in a chair.

In the following pages, we will take a detailed look at each of these massage therapies. Read on!

CHAPTER 7

Swedish Massage – For Relaxation and Wellbeing

Swedish massage describes a general massage system that uses a variety of techniques designed specifically for muscle relaxation and circulation.

By applying deep pressure to muscles and bones, the Swedish massage functions by rubbing in the same direction as the blood flows into the heart.

What are Swedish Massage's advantages?

A Swedish massage is a soothing and invigorating activity that enhances the supply of oxygen in the blood.

Through applying gentle but firm pressure, a Swedish massage can: enhance circulation, eases muscle pain, decrease muscle tension, enhances flexibility, induces relaxation, and Swedish massage promotes health and wellbeing in the skin, nerves, muscles, and drums.

Injuries such as muscle pain are used to shorten the recovery period of Swedish massage by flushing the uric acid, lactic acid, and other metabolic waste tissues.

Swedish massage increases circulation without increasing the heart load and extends ligaments and tendons, maintaining them soft and flexible.

A Swedish massage is ideal for physical and emotional stress reduction and can be used for a stress management program.

Swedish Massage - How Does it Work

The Swedish massage, invented in 1812 by the physiologist, Pehr Henrick Ling at Stockholm University, maybe the most common and widely known of all massage therapies.

The Swedish massage techniques include prolonged gliding strokes, kneading of individual muscles, rubbing, hacking or scratching, vibration and effleurage.

o Effleurage: palm, thumb and/or fingertip strokes

o Flapping: kneading movements with hands, thumbs and/or fingers

o Friction: round hands, thumbs and/or finger palm pressure

o Vibration: oscillatory motions shaking or vibrating the bodyshell: brisk hacking or tapping Passive and active movements: Bending and stretching every type of stroke of the body

Is Swedish massage safe for all?

Swedish massage is generally considered relatively safe. Some medical conditions, however, require caution. These include cardiovascular and cardiac conditions, especially in cases of thrombosis, phlebitis, and edema.

In the first 3 months of pregnancy, pregnant women should avoid acupuncture to the abdomen when the risk of miscarriage is greatest.

In case of doubt, please inform your doctor before seeking treatment.

Swedish Massage-What's going on in a session?

The body is wrapped in a blanket during a Swedish massage. The therapist detects one part at a time, massages the area before it is covered again and moves onto the next.

Oils and lotions are mostly used to promote relaxation with gliding and kneading strokes.

A Swedish whole-body massage usually takes between 60 and 90 minutes.

Swedish Massage–Choosing a therapist Based on your needs and preferences, Choosing a Swedish massage therapist.

A female therapist is preferable for both men and women.

People because they feel uneasy about another man's idea, and women because they feel safer to be a half-dressed woman rather than a strange man.

Salons, spas, health clubs, and exercise areas usually offer a Swedish massage or a Swedish massage can be arranged at home.

Brief Insight Into the Art of Swedish Massage

Massage is a technique used to relieve pain or discomfort for the patient. The massaging of the deeper functions and also of the surface layers of the muscles increases.

It also helps the connecting tissues to function better. It relieves the patient from pain or discomfort. There are different types of massage techniques and the Swedish massage technique is so common.

What is unique in Swedish?

Like any other form of massage, the Swedish approach is also based on strokes. A popular Dutch practitioner named Ohann Georg Mezger would have invented this Swedish massaging technique.

What is unique about the Swedish technique is the stroke type that is used for the disease. Kneading, friction, sliding or Gliding, rhythmic and vibration tapping are all types of strokes used in Swedish methods.

Swedish massage The technician will ask about the general health of the patient before the massage begins. He will also ask the patient about his allergic medication reaction. He will also ask if the patient has undergone any surgery or has been wounded. Only then will the massaging process begin.

The masseur shall exert enough pressure to prevent the patient from feeling uncomfortable. The masseur adds specially prepared oil to the patient's body before administering the stroke.

He should massage the oil on the body softly. This is a body lubrication operation. After the oil has spent some time on the body, the masseur performs correct strokes on the body.

When the stroke is administered, the body is warmed up. The muscles and the associated tissues are relaxed by warming up. It increases the blood circulation in the tissue and relieves the patient from pain and discomfort.

The strokes used in Swedish massage techniques are so powerful that even the muscle nodes can be broken down to provide the patient with much-needed relief. The duration and frequency of the massage depending on various factors, such as the patient's overall health, the severity and related factors.

The specially designed massage table

The massage is done on a massage table that has been specially designed. The table is designed to make the patient feel uncomfortable during the massage. The masseur then has the option to change the table height so that he can easily apply the strokes. Swedish massage techniques are used by most spas and massage centers across Europe

The Hallmarks of Swedish Massage and How Can It Benefit You

When people think of massage therapy, Swedish massage techniques are most likely. Yet what really is the Swedish massage?

Swedish massage is one of America's most common massage techniques, and if you're new to massage, it's a great entry point. The methods can be tailored for those who are pressure sensitive and for those who want deep muscle relaxation.

Different therapists may be specialized in massage styles, but there are a few common features that distinguish a Swedish massage from other forms of massage therapy.

Preparation, positioning, and warm-up You will generally lie on a table with your face in a U-shaped cushion for a Swedish massage so you can breathe easily without strapping your mind to one side.

It is often done with you nude or almost nude under a sheet. You can wear underwear, a swimsuit or a tank top and shorts if you want. The massage therapist will only remove those parts of the book at a time, depending on the part of the body. Most Swedish massage practitioners will start by using massage oil to warm your skin and relax your muscles.

The therapist will really reach in to relieve the nodes and stress once the muscles are slightly warm and supple. Many massages started with your back and followed by the back of your legs and the front of your legs, arms, and shoulders and, finally, your neck and your head.

Swedish massage methods Some movements and acts apply to Swedish massage. The word "effleuraging" refers to the movement of skin gliding and stroking. "Petrissage" refers to the kneading process that a massage therapist uses to dissipate nodes and stress in muscle meat.

"Tapotement" is a rhythmic tapping motion by the thumb, hand base, or back of the hand. A specialist may also use friction to generate heat, improve your circulation, stimulate your nerves, and relax your muscles.

Some masseuses also use vibration or shaking of some muscles to induce a more relaxed state. Which measures the massage therapist will take depends on your health and fitness levels, on the areas of your body that are feeling stress or sorrow, and on any massage objectives you have.

You may assume that a massage is meant solely to relax the body and reduce physical pain, but these are only two of the many benefits of a Swedish massage. Massage therapy can also increase your blood flow, reduce joint and nerve pain and enhance your lymph system.

In addition to helping to dissipate stress hormones, daily relaxation will help you sleep better. When gently and slowly applied as part of a managed physical therapy routine, Swedish massage can improve recovery time following a muscle or joint wound.

One of the great things about this massage is that it is easy to understand, even for massage novices. Unlike Asian massages based on meridians and energy therapy,

Swedish massages specifically concentrate on your anatomy. This makes adjusting the massage to your needs simple. Not sufficient pressure? Tell the therapist to dig more deeply.

If the therapist touches a certain muscle, does he experience pain? So she can adapt her work accordingly, let her know. When you feel nervous or uncomfortable with something, say so. The more comfortable and relaxed the treatment is, the better the performance

Swedish Massage in a Massage Chair Recliner

Over the years, massage recliners have evolved from basic vibrating chairs to luxurious massage chairs with fire, music and various relaxation therapies. The Swedish massage or classic massage is one of the most basic massage techniques. The Swedish massage was developed by Henrik Ling in the 18th century. Swedish massage is very efficient to absorb more oxygen in the body.

Most of us have tension in our everyday lives. At work, we may be under pressure that causes us mental stress. Mental stress leads to tension that doesn't relax the muscles. We should work out and do more physical activity. The muscles are tired and fatigue after they are under stress. The body can be influenced by both mental and physical stress.

Massage therapies have been developed and practiced over time to help alleviate pain, sadness, and sorrow. Swedish massage is one of the most common forms of massage. Swedish massage is intended to relieve pain and improve body health. This helps detoxify the body by increasing the metabolism of the cells, which reduces waste.

The Swedish massage uses 6 elements: effleurage, petrissage, friction, vibration, and traction. Effleurage uses long strokes that cover several parts of the body. Petrissage uses muscles to knead and pinch. Heat or pressure makes the muscles relax and blood flow.

Tapotement consists of clicking or cutting action to relax the muscles. Traction is the arms and legs pulling and stretching. Vibration is used to shake and relax muscles for stress relieving and capillary vessel stimulation.

Such six strategies are now incorporated into the best recliner for massage chairs on the market. In order to perform these massage techniques, these recliners use different mechanical components. Rollers are held out in the back of the chair and protect the arms, shoulders, and back.

Petrissage is performed in the pinching or kneading movement of the rollers. Friction is accomplished by applying heating elements to the chair to warm up body areas. The rollers perform a tapotement executing a rhythmic tapping motion.

The lower body uses the friction by manually elevating and lowering the footrest to reach the lower body. Vibration is carried out by positioning vibrating engines in specific chair locations.

All 6 techniques cannot be performed by all massage chair recliners. All methods are performed to different degrees and can vary between models and manufacturers.

The massage chair the Panasonic Real Pro Elite and Omega Massage Montage Elite have the widest range of these massage techniques. This Montage Elite is the most detailed Swedish because the Panasonic Real Pro Elite does not have full body control. Try both of them and make your own decision.

The Swedish massage came from Henrik Ling's day. Mr. Ling would be shocked that the technologies he pioneered today's robotic massage chairs were engineered. Many of the same advantages as his pioneering efforts can be found in these mechanical massages.

However, Mr. Ling discovered the real advantages of Swedish massage on a routine basis. Sporadic spa visits are not as effective as regular

requests. A massage chair receiver is a perfect way to perform routine if you are looking for Swedish massage techniques. The Swedish body massage is known as the treatment that many men and women undergo in the spa.

The idea was first conceived in Sweden and adopted in the United States, as you probably guessed. This is a simple but perfect massage method that benefits from kneading (like dough), rubbing with handles, fingertips, cuts and sometimes vibration (bowls and balls), which relieves the body and creates anxieties.

It'll be easy on your body and definitely shouldn't hurt. If you have issues with deep muscle pain, a Swedish massage procedure can be more effective than a repair massage after extra therapy is used to relax the muscles.

The methods used for the Swedish massage are supplemented by a number of health benefits. The treatment first calms a person and improves blood circulation throughout the whole body.

Your improved circulation leads to greater tissue oxygenation and more energy for you. If you have pain in your joints just like arthritis, a daily massage including the Swedish body massage will reduce discomfort and promote movement.

Massage therapy has a result that detoxifies the body. Stroking and pressure move poisons from your inner bodies and body tissue to the bloodstream and then remove them from your body. The elimination of toxins will reduce anxiety levels, typically lowering both blood pressure and heart rate in turn.

Also, the Swedish massage is done on a covered medicinal massage table for your personal comfort. A towel or sheet will cover your body apart from the region massaged at that moment.

A majority of your garments will need to be discarded for easy access and application of oils. Many people are shy about this and some don't know about it. Take your best decision.

The oils can be used to improve the way the massage therapist operates. When you feel discomfort at any point in time, make sure you let him know. The Swedish Rest Massage is certainly one of the most soothing and gentle massages you can have, so enjoy your experience. You can even play songs in the background or low lights to relax you further.

The Moves of Swedish Massage

Five forms of strokes consist of a Swedish massage. The first is a scrub that is nice long strokes with light pressure that heats up the muscles. This move is probably the most common when you think about a massage.

The next thing is petrissage. Petrissage is a scooping motion that affects the muscles and the fascia of the body. Fascia is the connective tissue surrounding the whole body. This gets tied or trapped and has to be loosened occasionally.

Vibration is another step. Vibration is the body's movement moving at its own pace. It feels very good and can really make you sleep.

Another move is known as friction. Friction is perpendicular to the muscle fiber or circular to the way the muscle fiber functions.

The final move is called tapotement and can be a movement like cupping, cutting, quacking or hacking and is probably the second most important move to remember when contemplating a massage. It can be pretty noisy, so it is not done long and typically at the end of the session because it allows the sleeping customer to get up.

Such movements are all part of the basic Swedish massage and can be used at any time by the massage therapist.

Flow Swedish massage flows at a good pace of relaxation. There are no hurry or rapid motions in this kind of massage except for the tapotement. The people receiving a good Swedish massage usually sleep easily. And snoring is the therapist's complement.

Benefits: hyperemia and redness of the skin or organs, enhancing blood flow that supports the body's metabolism, releasing endorphins from the amino acids that act as the body's naturally occurring pain killers, and eventually increasing immunity by stimulating the activity of the lymphoid, which forms part of the natural defense mechanism of the body.

Music

A Swedish massage typically also has a musical part. There is lovely relaxing music during the massage. The music varies depending on the massage venue. For example, a massage franchise plays the same company-approved music. In a private or community session, the therapist plays music or encourages the client to choose their music or to make their own CDs.

In a relaxing massage, lighting is an important factor. After all, when you have spotlights or those God's terrible fluorescent lights, it is hard to relax. Sidelights or lamps are a good light source as long as the lamps are dimmed. Although fire regulations can prevent the use of candles in an office building, some therapists can even use candles in their practice.

Improvements Other things may be added or added by the therapist for an additional fee such as aroma, Reiki, scrubs or wrapping, hot stones, and cup massages. All the components of a nice relaxing

Swedish massage is there. In the following chapter, I will discuss a therapeutic massage that uses deep tissue movements to carry out a massage primarily.

The Swedish massage is said to be the most basic method of massage. Swedish massage is intended to enable the body to absorb more oxygen and to speed up the cells' waste disposal and thus to promote detoxification.

Swedish massage mainly works with the body's muscles and connective tissues to enhance circulation and decrease discomfort. This type of massage reduces muscle strain recovery times by allowing lactic acid, uric acid, and other metabolic waste to be removed from the tissues.

The tendons and ligaments are also flexible and elastic because of their stretching. Swedish massage will also relax nerves and skin at the same time.

In Swedish massage there are 6 main techniques. These six techniques include effleurage, petrissage (passive and active movements), friction, vibration, tapot or percussion.

Effleurage is the use of palm, thumb, or finger gliding strokes. Blowing may give the sensation of the breakdown of muscles, but the object of blowing is to attach one part of the body to the other. The kneading of hands, thumbs or fingers involves petrissage.

Petrissage does not concentrate on any specific part of the body, but the kneading makes a deeper and intense effect on the muscles. Circular pressure is the friction of the hands, thumb or finger palms.

The heat produced throughout the friction cycle relaxes the muscles and is used primarily to heat the area with the target muscles. Vibration uses oscillatory motion which shakes or vibrates the body.

Vibration is carried out by pushing the hand's heel and sometimes the fingertips forward and back over skin to relax the targeted area's muscles. Percussion or taping requires destructive hacking or tapping. This approach helps to energize and calm the region being handled at the same time.

Percussion is often performed when you cut the area with your hands' sides or rhythmically strike the area with hands cupped or fisted. Traction involves pulling the customer's arms and legs, and sometimes the ears.

In Swedish massage, passive and active motions bend and stretch. Such exercises are always carried out at the end of the massage because if the muscles were not relaxed, it would be painful. Swedish massage is usually done with oils or lotions on bare skin and the customer is either partly or entirely dressed.

Swedish massage is primarily based on Western wellness and healing views, while other massages with the use of acupressure and the Chinese meridian system can focus on Eastern viewing. A Swedish massage is a great tool for physical and emotional stress removal.

It is recommended regularly as part of a stress management program. The Swedish model is a good place to start for those who receive their first massage because it is not too aggressive and relaxing.

CHAPTER 8

DEEP TISSUE MASSAGE

Deep Tissue Massage - Muscle Tendon and Ligament Relief

Deep Tissue Massage or myofascial release is a massage technique that focuses on releasing constraints in the deeper muscle, tendon and ligament layers.

Deep tissue massage releases chronic pain cycles into the body through gradual strokes and deep finger pressure to contract areas.

A deep tissue massage warms the soft tissue first, by applying slow strokes and intense pressure or friction through the grain of muscles not with the grain, before reaching for the lower muscle groups.

Massage of the deep tissue-How does it work?

The treatment of deep tissue is both medicinal and corrective. We use two approaches, direct or indirect, to release deep stress patterns, to eliminate contaminants, to relax and to relieve muscles.

The direct approach applies muscle pressure in order to locate resistance in the body and keep the pressure until resistance is released.

The indirect approach travels in the opposite direction.

The amount of pressure applied to both methods depends on the amount of resistance.

Fingertips, knees, hands, elbows, and forearms all have long, slow strokes.

Because of the focus on a specific area, deep tissue massage may be uncomfortable for some customers and cause some sorrow during and after.

In order to correctly conduct the massage, any soreness will vanish within a day or two.

Deep tissue massage doesn't have to be very hard and it doesn't have to be uncomfortable, and pressure may be ineffective if done incorrectly.

There are many different combinations of the two forms, direct and indirect.

Some of the better known are: Polarity Therapy or Thai Massage or Triggerpoint Therapy. What are the benefits of a Deep Tissue Massage?

Unlike a standard relaxation massage, a deep tissue massage effectively acts on the skeletal structures deep inside the body.

Many people are looking for a deep tissue massage to help treat paralysis, muscle, tendon and ligament injuries.

As muscles are strained, oxygen and nutrients are blocked, resulting in inflammation that creates toxins in the tissue.

Throwing down the scar tissue and crystallization by regulated manual manipulation loosens muscles, removes toxins and encourages blood and oxygen to circulate properly.

It is important to drink plenty of water after the massage to flush away the toxins.

The most important benefits for deep tissue massages include:

o Removal of barriers that cause muscle strain

o Enhances blood circulation, lymph, cerebro-spinal and interstitial fluids

o Can overcome several chronic sources of pain by removing deep-seated feelings that cause stress.

Deep tissue massage can be very effective, but how much can be done in one session must be practical.

Only ask for more motivation and assume that if the therapist is pushing harder enough, all stress becomes impossible within an hour.

Only a series of therapies can fix chronic knots and tensions which build up over a lifetime.

Some practitioners will provide guidance on a schedule, including exercise, body practice, relaxation techniques, and a daily massage plan.

Was Deep Tissue Massage Secure to All?

As with most massage therapies, deep tissue massage for certain individuals is not recommended.

Treatment of the blurred or inflamed skin, open wounds, tumors, recent fracture areas, abdominal hernias, rashes or skin disease should not be done immediately.

The procedure should also be avoided: o people suffering from cardiovascular disorders and heart disease, particularly in cases of thrombosis, phlebitis and edema

o Predominant women and people with osteoporosis should consult their physicians immediately after surgery o If your doctor recommends the Deep Tissue Massage-Choosing a therapist W immediately after chemotherapy or radiation.

Lounges, spas, health clubs, and fitness centers usually have a deep tissue massage, or you contact a mobile spa and have a deep tissue massage at home.

Deep Tissue Massage for Pain Relief

Deep tissue massage is a type of massage therapy that re-aligns the inner muscle layers and the connective tissue. Such type of therapy is extremely beneficial to tissue muscles contracting around the spine, lower back and shoulders. This reduces the steep neck and less pain in the back.

The deep-tissue massage therapist massage movements are close to conventional massage therapy. This unique massage therapy helps break the scar tissues and remove them. This focuses on certain areas where the quick strokes and the intense direct pressure will help relieve chronic muscle tension.

A person with chronic muscle tension and injury usually feels pain from adhesions which are strong, painful muscle and tendon bands. It is generally thought that adhesions obstruct circulation, cause pain and inflammation, thus restricting the mobility of an individual. Deep tissue massage is recommended as the doctor kneads the adhesions gently and reduces pain while helping to restore normal movement.

To achieve this goal, the deep tissue massage therapists frequently apply intense pressure or friction to the muscle's grain. Occasionally people feel pain and related discomfort during the massage. In such situations, it is best to tell the massage therapist about the pain and sorrow if it is beyond the range of comfort.

Although after deep tissue massage there is some stiffness or pain, the amount of discomfort typically decreases within a day or so. Often the massage therapist applies ice to the massaged area.

Deep tissue massage is used for relaxation as well. The therapy is beneficial to those recovering from sports, osteoarthritis, muscle spasms and postural problems in particular. People with osteoarthritis opt for this therapy since it is very effective and they often notice significant mobility improvements right after the massage.

Therapists use fingertips, knees, hands, elbows and forearms during deep tissue massage. During therapy, the doctor works on the muscle below the upper muscle layer, which is particularly effective for people with chronic pain.

Once the massage is over, it is recommended to consume plenty of water to flush out metabolism waste from the tissues. The person may want to breathe deeply at the beginning of a tissue massage because this action facilitates the process and relieves tense muscles.

Deep tissue massage may not be the best for some kinds of people, such as heart patients or chemotherapy patients. Even in patients with osteoporosis, it is advisable to consult the therapist beforehand. The massage therapist tries to relieve pain from deeper tissue structures and care may be more painful than the traditional massage.

Furthermore, when considering this massage therapy, people must be rational. The deep massage in tissue may not immediately relieve pain but many think that if the therapist kneads hard on the pressure knots, he will receive immediate relief.

This could not always occur, as it is better to remove chronic nodes and build up stress over a lifetime if the person goes to an intensive program that includes exercise, posture improvement, mobility improvement, additional techniques for relaxation and daily deep tissue massage therapies.

Such a duel program is very valuable for body alignment. If the deep tissue massage is done properly, the effects could be felt in the next few days.

Since tensed muscles trap oxygen and nutrients when creating muscle tissue toxins, this form of massage is recommended because it removes the toxin from the muscles while it is loosened, allowing blood and oxygen to better circulate.

The primary purpose of a deep tissue massage is to relax muscle fibers and release heavy stress patterns so as to relieve the tendon. The treatment of deep tissue massage is both corrective and therapeutic.

Low finger pressure and slow strokes on the spots are a blend of contact, biomechanics and positioning possibilities. The massage technique uses knuckles, palm, forearms, and elbows to help release pressure and tension from the body's deeper layers.

Using Deep Tissue Massage Therapy to Reduce Musculo-Skeletal Pain

Deep Tissue Massage is used regularly and focuses on the deeper layers of the soft tissues of the body. It is designed to release chronic stress cycles through deep pressure and slow strokes on the contracted area(s).

This massage therapy is both supportive and corrective, and should not cause excessive discomfort to the client or stress to the therapist properly. Deep working is not equated with working harder and harder but is due to specific techniques of deep-tissue massage combined with knowledge of the different layers of the soft tissues of the body.

It is a term that therapists often use to suggest that they use high pressure and not only massage oil onto the skin.

Deep tissue research is not only about the amount of pressure used; it is true to work on all the layers of the soft tissue of the body and particularly their structure-the Fascia. Injuries, diseases or prolonged immobilization can make fascia stiff, hardened or stuck in neighboring structures. This, in turn, causes pain, mobility and work.

While at times slightly uncomfortable, it should never be painful; a good massage therapist should always be mindful of your pain tolerance and work with you in order to find a safe level of pressure for you.

The methods of massage include knuckles, toes, elbows, and forearms. The rate of a deep tissue massage session is generally slower than that of another massage, enabling the therapist to collect information from the tissue of the customer, to assess the best way to respond to the tensions and contractions identified and to apply careful and sensitive pressure to achieve comfortable and lasting release.

How does it work?

Due to long-term muscular stress, postural imbalance, overuse and injury, pain and stiffness in muscles and joints may occur. All this can shorten muscle fibers, cause small pockets of scar tissue to form (fibrosis), and larger areas of scar tissue to heal.

Shorter muscle fibers often contribute to decreased blood flow to the area and inadequate removal by the lymphatic system of metabolic waste products.

Areas of soft tissue that become rigid, hard and "glued together" in contract bands-adhesion-are the net result. It is impossible to move normally, with discomfort and pain.

Deep tissue massage works by operating gently but firmly across these lines, re-separating the tissues, lengthening shortened soft tissue structures and facilitating effective circulation to and from the area affected.

Who Benefits from Deep Tissue Massage Therapy?

This form of massage is particularly useful for people with chronic muscle pain, especially in the muscles around their arms, lower back, and shoulders.

This can be caused by postural problems, recreational activities such as gardening, sports, and exercise-related injuries as well as the end of long-term emotional stress and stress.

• releasing tension and rigidity from muscles, tendons, ligaments, joints, and fascia

• pain relief

• increasing flexibility and flexibility

• disintegrating old tissue of the scar and adhesions· improved mobility, posture, and physical performance •

quicker, more efficient recovery from injury and surgery

What to expect during and after a session

It can be offered in combination with other massage styles, as a whole-body therapy or in one area, for instance, in the lower back or shoulders. Your therapist works with you to find a comfortable pressure level and works with your breathing to minimize discomfort and get your tissue released as well as possible.

In the next few days, when a deep tissue massage is done correctly, the benefits will come. Based on the therapy session, you can feel rejuvenated or a little sorrowful. Some residual discomfort or pain after a deep tissue massage is an entirely normal reaction and will reduce within 24-48 hours.

Following the tissue massage procedure, take a warm bath and drink plenty of water and/or grass teas to help the body absorb any waste products from the soft tissues. It is best to rest and relax as much as possible. For the same reasons, it is also recommended to avoid caffeine and alcohol.

While massages are typically comfortable, deep tissue massage remains the counterpoint when therapists throw away children's gloves and function like an unmolded dough pad. While a little pain or sorrow may occur after a deep tissue massage, it is a good way of releasing tension in the long term.

Deep-tissue massage is a massage style that focuses on relieving muscle tension below the top muscle surface, as well as fascia or body tissue tension.

A range of methods (including the use of the elbows, fingers, or wooden props in some cases) is used by the massage therapist to loosen hard-to-reach muscles and to relieve a high level of tension in order ultimately to realign deeper muscle and connective tissue layers.

In the case of muscles, tendons, or ligaments, adhesions (bands of rigid tissue) may be very painful, restricting mobility and blocking circulation. Deep tissue massage prevents these adhesions by direct deep pressure on the grain in the sore muscles in question.

It is generally defined by its slow strokes, i.e., it is by no means a fast process. Deep tissue massage is recommended to be administered regularly, in order to correct long-term muscle tension and to prevent injury.

Who needs it?

Deep tissue massage is usually suited to a specific problem, including chronic pain, limited mobility, injury recovery, arthritis, or muscle spasms. It is also ideal for stiff backs, lower back pain and sore shoulders. In addition, a therapist can only focus on one particular problem area in a session.

This treatment is rather serious, so you don't think you're going to sip on wheatgrass smoothies while wearing nice small robes and slippers. This is not to say that a patient must have a deep tissue massage for physical pain, since it is good for his overall health, in particular, the limb of his muscles.

The intense, sometimes painful massage can only be justified when you have a condition that requires immediate attention. People participating in heavy physical exercise, athletes for one or those in constant pain are the most likely to receive deep tissue therapy during multiple sessions.

Benefits

Though you may have some discomfort or pain during or after a deep tissue massage, it is a long-term benefit to your health. Luckily, any pain or sorrow that occurs usually reduces in a day, and then obviously, you will feel better than ever, provided that all of the intense stress is released from your core muscles.

Indeed, once you get used to intensive deep tissue massage techniques, you will most likely find it pleasant and relaxing. Overall, the muscles are very healthy because it releases toxins, prevents inflammation, and helps circulate the blood and oxygen more appropriately.

Risks

In addition to initial pain or discomfort, there are not too many risks to deep tissue massage unless your skin is the same as a plastic bag.

This means that this type of massage is usually not recommended for individuals immediately following surgery, pregnant women, or anyone who has infectious skin conditions, rashes, open injuries or abdominal hernia.

If you are prone to blood clots, you should also ask your primary health care professional before receiving a deep tissue massage, because blood clots are at risk of being broken during the session.

Finally you are not advised to eat a large, hearty meal prior to your appointment (so think first, if your massage therapist's office is next to an IHOP). It is often wise to remain hydrated, especially following the massage, in order to remove toxins from the body.

So if you thought about joining a combat club soon, you might want to stop there. Deep tissue massage may be the visceral experience you were looking for. And happily, it's safe for you, it's legal, and it doesn't need to reach a bunch of guys in the cellar. It shouldn't at least.

Massage Chair Performs Deep Tissue Massage

When you suffer from persistent, dull pain, muscle tension or chronic pain, a large number of regular massage techniques are simply not successful. In these situations, a deep massage of the tissue can exactly be ordered by the doctor.

A thorough massage of the tissue goes beyond the superficial layers of the muscles to the source of pain or discomfort. Muscles have long flexible tendons but may break and become shorter and less flexible, which causes pain and malaise. A deep tissue massage helps to stretch these tendons in order to restore their intrinsic strength.

During our daily life, our movements strain or stress our muscles and start to break down over time. Add damage to the equation and now add scar tissue, which again becomes less flexible.

Thus the massage has to penetrate deeply in the muscles to help break down the scar tissue and crystallize to obtain effective relief. Such deep penetration contributes to restoring muscle strength.

Professional athletes regularly receive deep tissue massages to strengthen their muscles, fractured scar tissue and improve mobility. This is particularly important after hard workouts and exercise.

Professional athletes are able to receive deep tissue massage therapy regularly and thus benefit fully from the treatment. Those of us who are not professional athletes are at a considerable disadvantage because we may not have a massage therapist available continuously.

Studies have demonstrated that deep tissue can relieve muscle pain, stress and anxiety. Because of the constant daily stress on our bodies, medications are only really effective if they are provided regularly and frequently.

A one-time treatment is not a one-time treatment. For daily pain relief, the adequate frequency must be provided. A deep tissue massage chair can be an immense help here. There is a wonderful range of potential massage therapies for pain relief areas.

Technology is still advancing rapidly and a deep massage of tissues has been incorporated into many of the leading massage chair brands.

Enterprises such as Panasonic, Omega Massage and others are pushing the limits of their chairs with increasingly diverse massage treatments. Such massage therapies include air compression, stretching, heating elements and, to name just a few, music therapy.

Software programs monitor the deep tissue massage in all its aspects. The program begins the massage more superficially and then it works gradually deeper into the muscles, creating strain, pain, and pain.

These massage chair companies develop therapies for people with more chronic conditions such as chronic pain, fibromyalgia, tightness, and even carpal tunnel syndrome. These areas are targeted by many new features.

For example, air compression massage offers airbags for your hands and forearms. The system must press, hold and release carefully. A gentle and repeated movement loosens the muscles, relieves pain and distress. Massage chairs can provide full neck to feet massages.

Deep tissue massage isn't for all. As this treatment is specifically aimed at hitting the deep muscle layers, most people can feel bad the next day. This is natural because the massage reached the deeper layers in order to relieve tension.

It is always advisable to ask your doctor if this type of massage is suitable for you if this is a concern. Many health professionals are optimistic that deeper tissue massage with more studies is shown to give chronic pain sufferers significant advantages.

Yet note, the effectiveness of massage therapy is routinely achieved. Stress, stress, anxiety are gradually increasing and must be constantly alleviated. Those with more chronic conditions should also be regularly treated with massage therapy.

As the damage to the muscles is more serious, the healing process takes longer. Seek pain relief. One great way to do this is to see which recliner for massage chairs are available. Every pain and every price range has one

How Does Deep Tissue Massage Differ from a Standard Massage?

Nearly every country has its own range of massages and each has its own uses and needs. Thai massages and Swedish massages, for example, are based on simple, but useful principles, which carefully work out the body and muscles. Indian massages following pregnancy have been designed to redistribute the fat of the body and improve muscle tone.

These simple massages are usually limited to the body's surface muscles and can be beneficial. Nevertheless, massage methods are developed for the care of the body, such as deep tissue massage.

What is the role of deep tissue massage?

Deep tissue massage is a somewhat different range of massages used to stretch muscle fascia.

They have medical value and are not standard practice recommended. As the treatment produces deep muscle bundles and ligaments, specific problems like osteoarthritis, muscle strains, fibromyalgia, back pain, repetitive strain lesions, etc. should be especially recommended

- The massage works on the body's connective tissue, which induces changes in the muscle tone and body posture. The massage procedure is designed to loosen layers of binding tissue not containing conventional massage techniques. The technique also releases underlying facial adhesion, chronic muscle contractions, tension, and muscle stress.

- Usually, five to six different strokes are applied to deep muscular bundles inside the body using the knuckles of the elbows, forearms, shoulders, ankles, feet etc. The velocity of the stroke is slower and pressured to ensure that deeper bundles of muscles are developed.

- Conventional massages will not cause body aches but are likely to cause muscle aches with deep tissue massage. One thing to note, however, is that pain levels vary from person to person. Many people find the process relaxing, but mild pains and soreness are normal.

These feelings are diminishing with time. You have to tell the therapist if you find the process uncomfortable and modify his strokes. Ice packs can also be used to relax the area immediately after a massage.

You may be perfectly healthy, but before starting treatment it is best to consult the physician. Deep tissue massage has many advantages, but it can also cause slight distress in deep-seated muscles.

This massage variation is not recommended for women with pregnancy, osteoporosis, diabetics, bleeding and coagulating disorders, etc. A complete medical examination and check-up are recommended before beginning any deep tissue massage.

The Health Benefits of Deep Tissue Massage

During one time, the idea of a massage brought a spa to mind. A luxury environment may come to mind in a health club or in a high-end resort. Deep tissue massage therapy has improved and so.

There are a number of types of massages. The overall term means skin, tendons, muscles, and ligaments to be manipulated and rubbed. Therapists normally rub their hands and fingers but also using the elbows and forearms to achieve the desired result.

Deep tissue massage requires a different technique. The slow and powerful method is used to reach connective tissue and muscle layers that are deeper in the body. This is typically the approach preferred to mitigate injury harm. Deep muscle massage focuses on realigning deeper muscle layers. The strokes are slower and deeper while many of the movements are the same.

While massages have in the past been considered to be an alternative kind of medicine, skilled treatments for a range of conditions and circumstances are increasingly popular. Those who subscribe to deep muscle massage will quickly tell you about their many advantages.

Deep tissue massage breaks down adhesions (rigid, painful tissue bands) and thus relieves pain and restores the natural movement of the customer.

The customer can feel some pain during the massage due to the pressure applied. The patient will warn the doctor if the pain or discomfort is beyond their own comfort zone.

Be mindful that you shouldn't eat a heavy meal before your appointment if you have never had a deep tissue massage. You will arrive 5 minutes early, so you can rest and relax a few minutes before the massage starts.

How to Choose Between Swedish and Deep Tissue Massage Therapy

There is a common misconception when it comes to massage that leads many to believe that one technique is very identical to another. It means that you often feel confused when they ask what kind of massage you are looking for when you book a massage.

You can choose the right type of massage because every type of massage therapy has its own advantages so it is important not to become confused. The Swedish massage and the Deep Tissue massage are two styles of massage therapy that are commonly mistaken for each other.

What is Massage in Sweden?

One of the most common massage therapies is the Swedish massage, consisting of a combination of kneading, pounding, gliding, friction, and vibration strokes.

The movements are normally used in a pattern that alternates between fast and slow strikes and different pressure levels. One of the main advantages of the Swedish massage is that the strokes supplement the normal blood flow to the heart and are effective for stimulating the lymph system.

Some of the advantages of regular Swedish massage treatments include improved blood circulation, loosening muscle tensions, increased relaxation levels and removal of metabolic waste.

During this kind of massage therapy, it is not uncommon for people to experience emotional release. Swedish massage is particularly popular in people with osteoarthritis or any kind of muscle pain or limited movement caused by old wounds.

What is the Massage of Deep Tissue?

Deep tissue massage therapy has been developed in contrast to research on connective tissue in the body. In contrast to Swedish massages, strokes are always done slowly in this massage style, although the pressure level can vary. If the strokes are done quickly, the connective tissue, also known as the fascia, is not adequately handled and the benefits are lost.

When used on a regular basis, deep tissue massage can help break down the old scar tissue and also encourage oxygenation in the body. That is why the massage of deep tissue is often marketed as good for the skin.

The strokes used in a deep-tissue massage are very similar to those used in the Swedish massage, where confusion originates, but the main difference is that the therapist is working against the grain of muscles when doing a deep tissue massage.

It is also common for instruments to be used during the treatment of deep tissue. These are either glass or smooth wood and are used in combination with wrists, elbows and fingers to optimize the therapeutic effects.

CHAPTER 9

WHAT IS TRIGGER POINT THERAPY?

Trigger point therapy is a physical therapy requiring muscle node massage because this helps relieve pain. The muscles in the spine, back and leg are the tightest knots in the body. Another type of treatment helps relieve stress in the body's muscles.

The aim of trigger point therapy is to remove the sore area rather than simply treat inflammatory pain on the surface. The trigger point therapy helps to identify and remove the pressure clusters, which can help eliminate pain.

The causes in the body cause serious discomfort, including hypersensitivity, muscle tension, muscle weakness, joint rigidity, numbness, stabbing and gunpowdering pain.

Dizziness and nausea can also be caused. The trigger point must, therefore, be removed to alleviate pain. Those who receive this massage can feel sorrow for several days after the session. Muscles should be stretched out often to keep the muscles from being locked again.

Massage trigger-point devices can be used to relieve muscle tension and excessive body pain in the comfort of your home. Every procedure relieves the muscles and stimulates points for different effects.

The Backnobber tool looks like the Thera-Cane but has its own useful features. For easy travel in a sleeping bag or suitcase, the rear nobber can be cut. The backnobber can be used by small and large people as well.

The Thera-Cane is the most common and powerful trigger-point massage device that can allow you to reach or reach all places in your hands.

It is important to stretch the muscles before using the Thera-Cane, as this helps to identify areas of tenderness. The rod is made of fiberglass and cannot be broken or twisted. The tool has no disassembly functionality like the Backnobber Tool.

The Lacrosse balls are the next useful trigger for therapeutic massage. Balls of lacrosse. Using them by lying against the wall with the lacrosse balls to penetrate the trigger points in the body.

These balls are made of rubber and have a better texture compared to tennis balls ' texture. It is similar to the Safe Body Ball Massager, but the lacrosse balls have a smooth texture around the ball.

The trigger points assist with various levels of pain. There are several different heads on the Pressure Pointer to detect distracting body pain. This offers immediate pain relief for every person who uses this drug. Pain relief and stress release from the pressure point is assisted by massaging the pressure points.

This tool has more extensions than the tools available for Thera Cane and Backnobber. The device has several rolling massage heads, adjustable properties and a foam grip which helps the massager use it.

Another effective massage device at Trigger Point is the Safe Body Ball Massager.

This is a round ball tool for convenience or the floor can help alleviate body pain. It can be used against a Lacrosse Ball-like wall.

This helps the body to alleviate pain and enhance blood circulation. The Safe Body Ball Massager seems to have these amazing circular fat spikes around the ball. The device is ideal for healing, enhanced joint or muscle strength, decreased muscle spasm, strengthened posture, alleviated tension, helped relax and shortened the pain cycle.

While in systemic health care the average individual is a bit confused, maintaining a healthy musculoskeletal system is an important part of healthy living.

Maintaining a good posture and strong muscle tone not only alleviates tension and pain but also improves the quality of life as the body grows older and succumbs to natural wear and tear. Structural health solutions like chiropractic or various massage techniques and soft tissue are available. Trigger point therapy (TPT) is a kind of gentle strategy, readily understood and can be performed by you or others. It is important to know first of all what a trigger is and how the TPT functions to better understand how you can benefit from TPT.

A stimulus is basically a region located in a muscle in which the muscle contracts or spasms on a small scale and forms a narrow "node" or muscle nodule.

Such small spawning areas are presumed to be the product of a chronically stressed muscle which seeks to conserve energy by increasing muscle fibers in bundles throughout the body. Trigger points may refer to other pain areas and different muscles have different pain reference patterns.

During Trigger Point Therapy, these nodular regions of a muscle strain are isolated. TPT can be performed manually or by specialized tools. The basic concept is to apply constant pressure for a short time to the trigger point, then release and repeat.

Several processes occur when the trigger point is pressured. The pressure breaks off the connection between the muscle and its underlying connective tissue, called fascia, so that muscle fibers can relax like a typical massage.

Nevertheless, the most critical mechanism seems to be the movement of the blood and the interstitial fluid (the fluid that surrounds all tissue cells in the body). When the pressure is released, the tissue fills in the field with fresh blood.

The media and discharge cycle for TPT basically flushes into toxins and by-products of the interstitial material from muscle cells and allows rich blood nutrients to rush in and help tissue repair and cure. It also begins to break up adhesion to the tissue. The end result of TPT is strong muscle relaxation.

TPT is most easily done on another person, but in other parts of your body, it can be done on yourself. Unfortunately, there will always be areas you can't reach, especially on your back! Fortunately, perfect trigger-point advice methods are available readily for "do it yourself."

TPT is an excellent way to improve your body. Read more about TPT in the Natural Health Portal. The natural health tool offers a free lesson on initiating point therapy that is easy to understand. We also provide TPT instruments and educational material services. Let the Natural Health System help you first in getting systemic health rights.

Trigger Point Therapy with Acupuncture Can Reduce Your Pain

Trigger Point Therapy is a chronic disease that causes muscle pain that can happen almost anywhere in the body. This form of pain may also be called' knots' or' spasms.' The word ' myofascial pain' may be used in the medical field. It means that the pain will occur in the muscle tissue and/or in the connective tissue around the muscles.

Eliminating the' knots' with acupuncture needles will quickly alleviate the trigger point pain by inducing relaxation or relaxation of muscle fibers that sometimes manifest as spontaneous twitches in the muscle tissue called vesiculation.

Pint pain cause can be chronic if left untreated. When left untreated for as long as possible, this pain will reduce the joint's or limb's motion. This stage is usually called "frozen." Even at this point, acupuncture is very effective in growing a join or limb's range of motion.

Another way to alleviate discomfort from trigger points is by using the "Balance System" of Dr. Richard Tan. This approach is based on the old Ba Gua numerology scheme. This method does not remove the trigger point locally but uses complimentary meridians, which are often distal or far from the pain site.

This technique is a highly effective way to reduce discomfort and increase the range of movement. If the acupuncturist does not want to stick needles in the muscle tissue itself, it is avoided because it is too painful.

Acupuncture Trigger Point Therapy is a faster and more often effective way of treating pain syndromes than manual or massage therapy. The healing process is usually longer and the acupuncturist can often penetrate deeper muscle and connective tissue layers.

Trigger Point Therapy - Knot to Be Overlooked

Trigger point therapy is a different form of massage, but it can go hand in hand, as part of the job of massage therapists is to relieve the stress that involves breaking up any sort of knot.

Trigger point therapy, as I first discovered this, was kind of upset because the student therapists working with me had difficulty finding trigger points. I think trigger point therapy was one of the most amazing things, now that I know what they are and how they feel.

I am a big man, I am very weak and I generally lie on my side with my hands in my ears as I sleep. This and some other that holding habits I have, like slopping and pulling to the body's front.

All of them have their own holding habits, which account for almost 99% of all muscle pain and some joint pains.

And yes, even Migraines can cause them.

Trigger points to me, feel like you're rolling over a little hardball or tendon when you massage, usually you can roll somebody's shoulder and feel a few of them.

Do you ever wonder, until you discover them, what to do with them? Perhaps you haven't, or perhaps you're curious now.

I'm about to tell you either way.

The way to treat these evil buggers is by applying ischemic pressure. In short, take your thumb and move it for about 20 seconds.

You want to wash out the toxins, think like a pimple or a zit. You first press or break the pimple, then you drain, drain or flush trigger points to move in a circular motion towards the heart.

In short, this is the whole basis for triggering large books about the subject, of course, but I like it simply.

Another side note if you wonder what the trigger point really is, there are a few hypotheses of what triggers it, but the thing is that it's just a stressful place, either because of an incident or because of some kind of pattern of help.

Clinical Trigger Point Therapy Benefits and history For decades, trigger point therapy has been commonly used even though it is not a part of conventional medicine. Also called myotherapy or neuromuscular procedure, the therapy involves using intense pressure to reduce discomfort and manage muscular spasms at certain "trigger points" within the muscles affected.

A trigger point is muscle fibers malfunction. The fibers are strongly contracted at the nerve / fiber junction of the innervating nerve. The malfunctioning of the nerve connection creates tension and discomfort in the muscle, or in other parts of the body.

The positions and related areas of reference for these malfunctions are consistent from person to person. The therapist exerts pressure on different points in order to better manipulate the transition, activate malfunctioning fibers and relieve pain and/or stress.

Some in the medical community start to recognize the importance of manual therapy. The experiences of patients with chronic pain have also changed greatly.

The cumulative benefits of this treatment go beyond pain alleviation. Such benefits include greater flexibility, increased breathing, better movement ability, decreased rigidity or stress in the muscles and fewer headaches.

Dr. Janet Travell and Dr. David Simons, the American physicians, are widely recognized for developing many trigger point therapy theories. With back pain, Dr. Travell treated US President John F. Kennedy, leading her to become her personal doctor.

Dr. Travell published volume 1 of the Trigger Point Manual, published a series of articles on the subject and subsequently continued working with her colleague Dr. Simons to write the second volume published in 1992.

Dr. Laura Perry and her husband Jeff Geanangel created the Institute of Trigger Point Therapy in 2001. Frustrated with the current state of the health sector, the two pursued an alternative option in a less formal setting for the general public which provided highly efficient clinical services.

Based on Drs ' work. Dr. Perry has developed Clinic Trigger Point Therapy Protocols and a program for training practitioners on this most effective treatment, Simons and Travell.

The philosophy of Dr. Perry is based on the premise that:

1. A massage is a pain.

2. To understand the massage, one needs to learn to "speak the language" of pain.

3. If one acts on this[pain] perception, the "call" is received and the pain stops.

Clinical Trigger Point Therapy is the implementation of Dr. Simons and Travel's peer-reviewed science, in combination with Dr. Laura Perry's real-world experience and further advancement to create a robust and effective physical pain management program.

.

Chapter 10

Aupressure Massage Therapy Restore Balance and Harmony

Clean the body with a massage of acupressure. The acupressure massage is based on the ancient Chinese acupuncture healing arts but without the needles. The acquisition is achieved by applying medium pressure on certain trigger points throughout the body.

A form of massage therapy stimulates the body's strength to boost the immune system's effectiveness and restore balance in the body. Today technology is being used to find and activate the acupressure points of your body in today's first massage chair brands.

Acupressure is a massage technique that lets the body release blocked energy centers. Science has confirmed the existence by various electric techniques of meridian pathways. Chinese medical arts recognized these meridian pathways throughout the body to hold energy.

We found that certain points or centers, causing the body to become out of control, might be hindered or blocked. The energy flow could be manipulated and restored by applying pressure to certain pressure points within the body. Research has now mapped the acupressure points of the body and identified over 350 body points.

Acupressure massage is achieved with methods of kneading, rubbing and vibration massage. These massage techniques are used in tandem with the stimulation of acupressure points throughout the body.

The massage by acupressure is carried out by fast circular motions with medium pressure at specific trigger points. During the massage, the trigger points are stimulated to release blocked energy. The balance of energy is restored and the body is stabilized.

Massage acquisition therapy has many positive advantages. This helps relieve fatigue, muscle tension, pain, and soreness. It helps to harness the recovery powers of the body. The stimulation of acupressure helps to spread toxins in the body. As toxins build up in the body, the muscles become rigid. This muscle rigidity imposes pressure on the circulatory and lymphatic systems. It creates undue pressure on your body, which brings it out of balance and harmony.

Massage chairs use advanced technology to identify the trigger points of the body accurately. The software programs draw up a map of the users. The acupressure massage is then individually tailored for each user.

Alone in the back, there are almost 100 trigger points. Massage chairs will raise the acupressure points and apply massage techniques such as kneading, tapping and vibration. These massage treatments alleviate soreness, discomfort and soreness of the back, shoulder and neck.

Most manufacturers have developed air compression devices for the lower body. The air compression systems provide airbags with different nodes equipped for trigger points in the lower body.

The airbag inflates and drives the node into the trigger point when the air compression device is triggered. These are usually found on the back of the calves and on the base of the feet. The activation of these trigger points causes complete relaxation of the body and reduces accumulated stress.

New studies of acupressure massage show that this can help to reduce headaches, insomnia, dizziness, digestive disorders, constipation and even motion sickness in some cases.

We have just begun to understand the influence of acupressure recognized in China for centuries. Modern technology is used in the best recliners for massage chairs to provide more effective treatments for acupressure.

The true quality of the acupressure massage is often performed. Remember that stress accumulates every day, so stress should also be regularly released. The most cost-efficient and comfortable way to receive the advantages of acupressure massage is by using massage chairs.

Massage Chairs Incorporate Acupressure Massage Therapy

Massage of acupressure is an ancient art of healing. Can acupressure use pressure on the body's points of acupressure? The goal of acupressure is to control energy flow across the body. This helps to return the body to its natural balance. This ancient art of healing has been technologically advanced and is now available in the finest massage chairs.

The typical trigger points of the body are based on different forms of acupressure. The patterns, methods, and forces used are the variations between the forms. Shiatsu, for example, is a type of acupressure massage and its best-known form.

Some strategies involve applying firm pressure on trigger points for 3 to 5 seconds. Another technique involves the use of an occasional tapping pressure. Another technique involves steady pressure on the trigger points to calm the entire body.

Many of the best brands of massage chairs such as Panasonic, Omega and Sanyo include a body scan system to recognize precise points for specific individuals. The app then changes each person's massage.

There are more than 300 acupressure points throughout the body. These trigger points are used by acupressure to control energy flow throughout the body and to eliminate blockages.

The massage chair performs an individual scan and then the massage will reach the trigger points on the back, depending on the acupressure system. Many chairs use gradual kneading with firm pressure.

Some chairs use gentle light pressure, quick tapping. The programs in different model chairs can also vary from manufacturer to manufacturer. The best thing is to try some massage chairs to find out which ones are right for you.

To help you relax some massage chairs, the acupressure massage is complemented with other features. Most spas have soft meditative music to help the mind relax and avoid the stress of the day.

Some massage chairs are fitted with MP3 players and headphones for relaxation. Therapy can also be found where heating elements are built into the chair. Temperature leads to swelling and blood flow loss.

The acupressure massage supports blood and lymph flow. The increased blood and lymph flow increases energy and helps the body cure. In addition, some benefits of acupressure massage are as follows:

Blood pressure reduction in tension and anxiety

Increased awareness and alertness

Increased energy

Massage has been used in many ancient societies for centuries. Now technology has made both cost-effective and affordable acupressure massages with massage chairs.

In fact, massage chairs are a very economical way to achieve acupressure massage. The true advantages of acupressure massage are obtained daily. Like any procedure related to health, it needs to be done over time. With a massage chair recliner at home, you have exposure and a low-cost way of daily acupressure massage.

Contrary to certain forms of massage therapy, acupressure massage is part of an old Chinese medicine program designed to help relieve pain and promote natural healing by means of non-invasive bodywork.

Acupressure massage is based on "meridians" or canals that carry energy across the body. Prospective students will soon learn that acupressure massage correlates with acupuncture points; instead of using a needle, students will learn how to use gentle but firm hand pressure to produce the same results effectively.

In an acupressure academy, learners who learn how to perform acupressure massages will find that stress and stress relief, mind-body relaxation, enhanced circulation, musculoskeletal pain relief, and many other positive health effects are all important benefits of acupressure massages.

As well as insight into how acupressure massage leads to overall health and well-being, acupressure massage students learn fundamentals of acupressure, kinesiology, anatomy, and physiology as well as a variety of related Chinese medical studies.

Many massage therapy schools offering a massage of acupressure that teach students to use this specific bodywork in combining reflexology, aromatherapy and essential oils. Acupressure massage courses may also include seminars on Tui Na (Chinese Medical Massage), Zen Shiatsu, sports acupressure and specialized training on certain human and animal diseases, such as cancer and arthritis.

A number of natural healing schools expanding acupressure massage instruction can also provide courses in Qigong, Asian bodywork and other massage techniques.

As with most massage treatments, acupressure massage is an excellent addition to all the customer services provided by licensed practitioners. All students and practitioners receive a fair amount of training and improved training if they choose to enroll in this specific course.

Points, Sports, and Acupressure Massage

There are hundreds of massage therapy styles and techniques. Sometimes it's difficult to know what you are and what you are doing. It is difficult to ask for some form of massage if you don't know what it is called or what it will do for you. Here we try to break the mystery into an accessible list of certain massage styles and what they do.

The belief that the body is out of balance due to warped force, centered on unseen paths in certain points called meridians, is behind Shiatsu and acupressure.

Shiatsu is the term Japanese: the finger is the word "shi," and the pressure is the word "atsu." Shiatsu uses rhythmic pressure from 3 to 10 seconds in specific points along the meridians of the body by opening up feet, hands, elbows and knees and increasing the flow of energy. Oriental finger massage methods, such as acupressure and Shiatsu, treat acupressure points to relieve pain and restore strength.

Sports Massage

Sports Massage is targeted at all styles of sportsmen, from foreign athletes to casual joggers. It is a special form of massage and is used before, during and after sports. Sports therapy may help prevent those sniffing accidents, which so often hinder performance and outcomes whether an athlete or a jogger once a week.

It is designed to address these particular problems and can vary depending on the sport that athletes play. Sports massage can help to cure tight muscles and allow healthy individuals to achieve high performance while minimizing the risk of injury.

The pre-event, after-event and rehabilitation techniques can be used to promote improved sports stamina and performance, minimize injury opportunities and reduce recovery time. Not only does sports massage reduce heart rate and blood pressure, but it also increases circulatory and lymph fluid, reduces stress in the muscles, increases strength, and reduces pain.

Acupressure is practiced over 5000 years ago. It is a bodywork based on traditional Chinese meridian theory where acupuncture points are shifted in order to induce the energy or flow of Chi. The approach is based on acupuncture concepts. During acupressure, the palm, elbow or different instruments apply physical pressure to acupuncture points.

The therapist uses pressure to release small knots of contraction. This is activated by acupressure to eliminate barriers, increase energy transfer and promote health and harmony in the body. Shiatsu is the most popular acupressure form and Zhi Ya is a Chinese acupressure massage.

Reflexology

Reflexology is a method of hand and foot acupressure. It is a type of bodywork based on the theory of zone therapy where certain parts of the body are stimulated to stimulate appropriate regions in the body. Reflexology is a scientific foot massage based on the assumption that the feet reflect a "mini plane" of the body and that every corporeal and organ component is a football ground.

Reflexology uses pinpoint pressure and gentle strokes to help balance the body. Reflexology reduces pain, increases circulation and encourages the body's natural remedy. A reflexology session is intended to interrupt the stress cycles in the body and provide an overall relaxing feeling.

Effectiveness of Acupressure

The use of fingertips, hands, elbows, or feet to put pressure on the most important cures in the human body activates the body's natural self-healing abilities, which can be referred to as acupressure. It is an ancient Chinese healing art that was reported over 5000 years ago in Asia.

Acupressure therapy has been shown to be very helpful in the treatment of many stress-related diseases. Acupressure can actually reduce tension, alleviate pain, increase the circulation of the blood and increase overall health. Apart from treating stress-related conditions, acupressure is also used to rebuild reproductive cells, detoxify the body and boost the tone of the skin.

Acupressure therapy can help increase tolerance and prevent unwanted diseases of the body. Such treatment can be achieved by studying various techniques and conditions, such as muscle pain, mental stress, learning disabilities, emotional trauma and many more.

How will this work?

During the acupressure sessions, you are told to lie on a massage table (your clothes must not be removed). The nurse then starts to massage and rub the remedies gently. Every session can last approximately an hour. You need to attend multiple sessions to produce the best results.

The true goal of acupressure or any bodywork is to improve your overall health by controlling the negative and positive energies in your body. Most people believe that acupressure cannot only heal the body but also mind, emotion and spirit.

There are too many points of acupuncture in the human body to list. Nonetheless, the main points used by practitioners in the field of acupuncture and acupressure are large intestine 4 (Li-4). Acupuncture and acupressure are in the thick flesh between the forefinger and the thumb to treat large intestinal diseases.

Liver 3 (LR-3) Lip diseases are treated between the big toe and the second toe with acupressure and acupuncture.

Spleen 6 (SP-6) Acupuncture and acupressure are applied over the ankle at a limit of three finger widths for treatments of hepatic disorders. In the lower calf muscle, this area is very tender.

Who can benefit from acupressure?

Although many believe that acupressure can cure many problems, it is important to realize that the procedure and its ability to improve various health conditions are still not completely demonstrated.

This approach is a new treatment and further research needs to be done before all claims like, "acupressure is going to effectively treat such a disorder for many weeks."

Nausea and vomiting: A number of studies have shown that wrist acupressure can effectively treat nausea and vomiting, caused by several factors like post-operative pain and nausea Muscle sickness Pre and post-operative nausea, there are a little but complete reports of the following health conditions. PC 6 is the point of acupuncture and acupressure for the treatment of nausea and vomiting from the palm base between the two nerves. Specially designed bracelets that can track this medical condition are also in the medical counter.

According to various individual reports, cancer acquisition relieves stress, reduces stress, increases energy and decreases the pain in cancer patients, as well as eliminates nausea after chemotherapy.

There is some preliminary evidence of the effect of acupressure on lower back pain, trauma and headache. Specific pain: Acupressure can also improve diseases caused by other medical conditions.

For headache, the healing point arthritis is under pressure: the studies show that acupressure in arthritis patients can reduce inflammatory sensations in the joints significantly.

The medical explanation is that the application of acupressure releases endorphins that can trigger anti-inflammatory effects in the articulations and therefore reduce pain in arthritis patients.

Depression and anxiety: numerous studies show that acupressure can effectively reduce fatigue, depression, fear and improve the mood of an individual.

Precautions Acupressure is generally a healthy treatment. However, patients with health conditions such as cancer, diabetes, heart disease or any other chronic illness should consult their doctor before undergoing this treatment. Purchase is just a precautionary measure.

While acupressure therapy is still in its infancy, the majority of people who obtained it are pleased. This is certainly one of the best treatments for so many people, but the only downside here is that it needs to be done under the guidance of a licensed acupuncturist. Have good acupressure!

Acupressure Therapy - Health in Your Hand and Feet

Acquisitions Therapy was identified in India five thousand years ago, although it was not correctly maintained and in Sri Lanka's (Ceylon) form of acupuncture. Buddhist monks or nomadic Aryans from Sri Lanka brought this practice to China and Japan, and China teaches acupuncture worldwide now. This technique was studied by Red Indians in the sixteenth century.

In the 20th century, research was carried out in the United States, which significantly contributed to the advancement of this procedure. The most allopathic and naturopathic doctors are used but this simple and easy procedure has also been taken care of by the World Health Organization.

The word "acupressure" means "acupuncture" that involves a needle and a point to be crossed. The way to treat diseases is by perforating certain points in the body acupuncture. Acupressure means the art of treating diseases by applying pressures to certain areas, using thumb, figure or jimmy (wood or rubber stick).

Goal The goal is to promote the body's own healing power. Once the principal point of acupressure is placed on the surface of the skin, muscle tension is released and the energy of life of the blood and body which the Chinese call energy "chi" is stimulated.

Acupressure can be used to treat a variety of conditions, including everyday stress, fatigue, soreness of the neck and shoulder, pain, asthma, menstrual problems, fatigue, fearfulness and back pain, etc.

Precautions Acupressure for other medical conditions, such as severe burns, ulcers or illnesses should not be used. Be careful when using abdominal pressure points, especially when the patient is diseased and when a life-threatening disease like intestinal cancer or pregnancy is in the abdominal area, is avoided.

Acupressure usually uses thumb pressure, fingertips or jimmy acupressure devices. Blocking energy in these meridians can lead to physical discomfort, pain, stress, and tension.

The stimulation points remove the blockage of muscle relaxation and allow blood to flow more freely. It also releases an emotional barrier by releasing stress. The pressure can also release lactic acid which builds up in muscle tissues.

Throughout intense muscle activity, lactic acid is developed and is usually removed from the blood by the liver. It can build up in the muscle, however. There are different acupressure techniques in the west, including aqu-yoga: a whole-body technique that extends and the yoga positions push the meridian channels and trigger them.

Jin Shin Jyutsu: A self-help method of acupressure requiring a soft touch of the body rather than massage.

Do-In: a self-acupressure program that involves massaging meridian points and muscles and requires deep breathing, relaxation and exercise.

Shiatsu: a rigorous technique that involves the rhythmic rubbing of acupressure points.

Light to medium pressures are applied to acupressure points and rotated in a tight circle during acupressure. It's mainly done with your fingers, thumbs and palms. The elbows or knees are also used in the key pressure points. Because the most sensitive or critical points are pressed, the response helps to determine the right spot.

If the answer cannot be felt, the location of the pressure point may not be right, or the pressure may not be intense enough. The feeling should be in an acupressure session somewhere between pleasure and pain.

Three times the benefit of acupressure: therapy: the fast and accurate diagnosis— medical test without study.

Treatment: treatment for all types of diseases, including brain and cancer disorders.

Prevention: heart disease, paralysis, and cancer are all forms of disease prevention.

The world could be divided into about 60 percent from the perspective of well-being–all the stable yet disease-prone (including the born). There are many specialists and hospitals worldwide who can look after these men. Acupressure therapy can also prevent them from falling ill subsequently.

Risks: while acupressure can and should not be used as a replacement for traditional treatment, it can also be paired with other forms of treatment.

"Acupressure therapy is the most valuable gift of the creator himself"

Benefits of Receiving Acupressure Treatments

Acupressure is now an art that everybody knows. The real acupressure technique was to push and pressure the five specific points known as acupressure points to assist the different functions of the body.

Acupressure is believed to be a means of treating various health problems by pressure at certain points known as pressure points. The best thing about acupressure is that it is easy to learn and implement. There are three main advantages of individual acupressure treatments. There are few organs to rely on to gain the advantage of acupressure.

The first one among the organs is Large Intestine. This organ has acupressure points between the thumb and the forefinger.

The liver is another organ whose health would benefit from acupressure. This organ has acupressure points between the second toe and the big toe.

The next organ of choice is Spleen. This organ has an acupressure point over the inner knee of the lower calf muscle.

Use the listed stress points to relax the body for some time, maybe 5-10 minutes a day. Best results are achieved when the procedure massages all sides of the body. There are many benefits of acupressure therapy. The pressure points must be correctly positioned and the pressure applied in order to prevent the maladministration of the muscles.

Books are available that help a person learn more about the exact points of pressure and how to find the exact points of pressure so that acupressure treatments can benefit. The books usually show the pressure points pictorially so that the user can easily identify the pressure points.

It is, however, often best to visit an acupuncturist before the acupressure process actually starts, because he would be better able to guide a person about using the right methods and movement at the above-mentioned stress points.

Acupuncturists are individuals who are skilled in the practice of acupressure healing and have a thorough knowledge of acupressure theory and the associated stresses.

We are the only people who know what the competitive incentive to apply to a certain environment and for a particular benefit would be. An acupuncturist who has practiced the therapy for many years can explain well the benefits of acupressure treatment.

Some conditions are not recommended for acupressure. It is therefore absolutely essential to consult an acupuncturist before beginning acupressure therapy for health benefits.

Books may contain basic science behind effective acupressure treatments, but only an experienced acupuncturist would be able to perform the same procedure on the same pressure points to produce a particular benefit.

Acupressure is definitely an efficient way of treating a healthy lifestyle, but it should be performed under an experienced acupuncturist.

Chapter 11

Reflexology

What Is Reflexology?

Reflexology is an old, natural healing process that dates back at least 5,000 years to Egyptian and Eastern cultures. Many terms related to acupuncture are guided by special points and target areas as practitioners of both therapies.

Nevertheless, acupuncture requires the use of fine nails throughout the body, but meditation does not use needles and focuses on the feet. Reflexology can also be performed on the hands and ears.

Reflexological science considers the feet to be a mini-map of the human body with each organ, gland and part of the body linked to a specific reflex region or level of the foot. Reflexology speeds relief to a specific area or point for the appropriate part of the body.

A reflexologist can help heal individual conditions through different pieces of the feet, but it is desirable to work in all areas in order to balance the entire body. Some reasons for how reflexology tends to mitigate or reduce pain and distress are as follows:

Diseases: menstrual cramps

The area(s) of your foot should be treated by a reflexologist;

ankles top of the feet with inner skin related to the body of the foot

: reproductive organ conditions

: back, foot shoulder and neck stress

In addition to the actual registration of the foot stress

It increases the body's strength and energy, increases efficiency and creativity and offers an emotional balance. Clients with chronic problems, such as asthma, drug shortages, and weight management concerns, have also improved substantially.

Should reflexology be a medical therapy? No.

Neither medical nor foot massage is reflexology. Reflexology is a distinct form of natural healing. It is a science that involves research, sound technology, practice and patient art.

A person rarely feels pain during a reflexology session. There are 26 bones, 56 ligaments, 38 muscles and 7,000 nerves per foot, so many places are activated during a session. In a reflexology session, the sensations are felt in the feet not in associated muscles, glands or parts of the body.

But a client often feels sore 1-2 days after a session in various parts of the body. The explanation for the discomfort is that toxins are released from the feet during a session and often the physical removal mechanism takes some time to remove them. The open dialog between the client and the therapist is encouraged to take advantage of the session.

Reflexology is so strong and quickly taught. It has become so popular in recent years that it has been used as an additional tool by physicians, chiropractors, podiatrists, dentists, nurses, mothers, physical therapists, laboratory therapists, and massage therapists.

Imagine the following scenario to show how medical practice can be employed: a pregnant woman is put to work. Although her pain with modern pharmaceuticals can be treated, her lower back and neck still have pain and discomfort.

Reflexology is done on her feet, particularly on the inner edges, to help her alleviate pain in the back and neck. There are no pins, and there is nothing to reveal her foot. Within just an hour she experiences a new feeling of calm and the pain of her neck and back has gone, allowing her to focus on the miracle of childbirth!

Most inspired laypeople actively prefer reflexology to lead to raising stress in the lives of their friends and family.

Is reflection safe? Safe reflexology and daily sessions served people of all ages, including children and the elderly, and under numerous chronic conditions including diabetes, cancer, addictions, terminal disease and obesity.

Reflexology - The Art of Foot Massage

Reflexology is a supplemental treatment to help and relieve pain by operating on the feet in the other part of the body. Reflexology is a gentle treatment that helps restore and maintain your body's natural balance.

Reflexology cannot treat and do not claim to cure, diagnose or prescribe serious or life-threatening medical disorders but is highly popular with people of all walks of life as an alternative healing device.

Who can benefit from reflexology?

Reflexology is for all.

Many people are reflexology as a way of relaxing their minds and bodies. It has proven to be a useful tool for: o conditions of stress, o sleep disturbances, o back pain, o migraine or infertilities, or for sleep disorders or digestive disturbances, o hormonal imbalances or arthritis.

How does reflexology function?

Reflexology enhances mobility by relaxing and exerting pressure on your hands and feet and can facilitate different muscle and body functions.

Stronger hands and feet than most people know. A professional reflexologist can recognize subtle changes in certain points in the feet and, by operating at those points, may influence the associated body organ or device.

Reflexology has been shown to improve physical and emotional movements, enhance self-esteem and trust and promote motivation and concentration.

Which occurs in a reflexology session?

According to Chinese medicine, the feet's sole comprises the sensory nerves of the inner bodies dispersed across the body. In a reflexology session, the therapist puts physical pressure on the feet and focuses on specific areas that communicate with different areas of the body.

The pressure is then added to some parts of the sole of the feet. Deposits and imbalances are observed and discharged in order to remove barriers and recover blood and energy.

Reflexology uses hands, feet, a wood stick, cream and oils to cause certain areas to represent. Reflexology offers the body a sense of well-being and relaxation to help cure it if well done. You'll wear comfortable, uncontrolled clothes because only your shoes and socks are gone.

Was reflexology healthy for everyone?

If you have heart conditions, diabetes, asthma, high blood pressure, or kidney disorders, you should consult a healthcare professional before beginning a reflexology course.

Reflective therapy cannot be offered for 45 minutes every day if women and men who bleed internally or externally. You should start to experience a positive difference after one or two treatments. Many people feel relaxed and comfortable.

Often people report feelings of nausea, tearfulness or lethargy after a reflexology session. This, say therapists, is part of the healing process. It is important that you inform your reflexologist in order to follow your treatment plan.

Reflexology should be stopped at least one hour after meals. Like most massage treatments, you can drink plenty of water after treatment. Many people use meditation in order to calm their minds and bodies, which has become more popular in recent years to relax and relieve every day the pressures we face.

You can look for a properly trained therapist to get the most out of a reflexology session.

Most spas, salons, and centers now offer massage treatments and reflexological treatments are carried out at home by some therapists.

Reflexology Is Much More Than Just a Foot Massage

There are so many people who regard reflexology as a foot massage and nothing else. Let me illuminate you if you are one of these people.

The following paragraphs will discuss and explain reflexology. If you are looking for information that clarifies the numerous myths regarding reflexology, you are on the right path.

Reflexology is a procedure where a trained therapist uses thumb and finger pressure to point at his or her head, feet or even ears. Such regions are the body's trigger points. These reflex points connect to certain parts of the body and are carefully removed if the pain relief or imbalance in this specific area is massaged.

If your body system does not function properly, calcium, minerals and uric acid deposits can form in the reflex points which eventually interfere with the proper blood circulation. A professional reflexologist can use massage techniques to break down these deposits and help restore normal working conditions.

In fact, studies have demonstrated that 75% of diseases and disorders are caused by stress. The first thing you can do to stop stress-related diseases is rest and relaxation.

This is where reflexology begins. Concentrate on relaxation points will help your body relax by normalizing blood flow and relaxing the nerves, allowing the body to benefit more from reflexology.

There are numerous nerve endings in your hands and feet that are all connected to various parts of your body. You can stimulate the affected areas in your body once you locate and massage the right areas of your feet or hands.

While reflexology can be applied to the hands, most reflexologists prefer to treat the feet since they are larger and more comfortable to massage. For this reason, most people mistake reflexology as a foot massage.

Hand reflexology is great for patients who don't like to touch or look at their feet, and it's perfect for people who complain about hand discomforts like arthritis or carpal tunnel syndrome.

The reflexology applied to your hands can be carried out wherever you want without feeling uncomfortable and uncomfortable. But, because the hands are often overused, they can become less flexible and sometimes impair the efficacy of this kind of reflexology.

More and more people are changing into alternative treatments, including reflexology, in this time and age, because it does not guarantee any secondary effects. Reflexology can take several treatments until you feel the effects, but you will soon realize that they are really useful and highly effective.

If you want to know where and at what point reflexology are available, reflexology pictures and diagrams. Nonetheless, if you want an in-depth instruction in reflexology, you are highly recommended to join a reflexology program or course.

You can try your own skills, but when applied by another person, reflexology is better because you can relax more which helps the body's healing energy to be stronger. There is plenty of content to help you gain knowledge of the right points and pressure in reflexology or to help you obtain information for home therapy or for your own personal sessions.

Nevertheless, if you want to make professional use of your knowledge and training, your family and friends should start reflexology.

This serves two purposes; it teaches them the benefits of reflexology and helps you to gain experience and feedback. Recall that only when reflexology is properly done, make sure that you don't try without appropriate research and training.

Reflexology has long been misunderstood but is finally recognized not just like a foot massage. The research behind the procedure is well documented and positive results are well recorded.

Reflexology for the Feet

The reflexology of the feet, the legs, the face, and even the ears can be achieved! Foot reflexology is the most common, which many reflexologists believe is particularly suitable for treatment due to feet's sensitivity. Clients can use hand reflexology exercises in treatments as' homework.'

Reflexology is torture when you are very rarely ticklish! As soon as you relax you will find that the therapist's firm, sure touch does not tickle. I never lost a customer, since they find the treatment ticklish and many people were extremely pleasantly surprised.

My feet look awful, the reflexologist will comment upon them and embarrass me Before a treatment starts, a reflexologist will look at your feet.

When you believe that a chiropodist or a doctor needs treatment for a foot problem, for example, verrucas or maize, they'll tell you. Besides that, they're there to do a job and don't judge your feet. Your feet have a form and structure of their own and you have nothing to be ashamed of.

They're not too new after a day on my feet!

Also, there's not the reflexologist to judge you. We all lead busy lives and before your appointment, there is not always a chance to wash your feet. Most reflexologists will refresh the customer's feet before treatment begins.

Reflexology will tell you what's wrong with me and then heal me Reflective scientists aren't qualified to diagnose and don't assert medical treatment. We don't have medical training and that's the job of your doctor, in any case.

After all, reflexology supports your body, mind, and emotions naturally, and allows them to heal themselves, and there can be amazing results.

Reflexology is the technique to apply moderate pressure in reflex points of the hands and feet to achieve a deep relaxation state, to enhance the body's healing process and help a person return to a state of well-being and equilibrium (homeostasis).

What is reflexology doing for you?

Through each brain, glans and body system, a reflexology procedure operates. The many advantages it offers include rest, pain and stress relief, better circulation and digestion, stimulation of the nervous and immune systems and equilibrium between spirit, body, and soul.

Reflexology is a holistic approach as the whole person is treated rather than the symptom. Migraine, sinus problems, PMS and hormone problems; pregnancy, fertility and menopause-related problems; back, and joint pain; and insomnia, are just a few of the reasons reflexology may help to alleviate digestive disorders, such as irritable bowel or acid reflux.

Reflexology is not a magical cure, but I saw some amazing results after a few treatments. How quickly you respond to reflexology is dependent on all sorts of factors, such as the duration of your life. In general, we expect to see some healthy and well-being results after 4-6 sessions, and it is typically best for the treatment plan to continue with weekly treatments.

How can I make the most of reflexology?

Your body is a little like a car–if you love and respect it, have it washed and served frequently, give it water and oil, and practice the right safety controls, it should be of good service to you for years. I always find that reflexologists are the people who have put in a little effort to improve their general well-being and wellbeing.

Your reflexologist will explore your lifestyle in detail, and together you can find things that can help you improve your health. These could include drinking more water, reductions in caffeine, a more balanced diet, getting food advice, looking for ways of improving your health, or finding ways to relax and reduce stress.

When you go to reflexology, what happens?

To have reflexology, you don't have to dress just to remove your socks, shoes, and shows. Men may want to loosen their tie, and for their comfort straight belts can be removed. Ladies have to remove their clothes or shops. You sit on a special chair or lie on a sofa after a consultation with your reflexologist.

This position allows you to be comfortable and your feet to work with the reflexologist. After a relaxing foot, he or she normally works in a special sequence one foot at a time.

The fingers and thumbs of the reflexologist work around your feet gently, pressing your thumb and using other techniques to stimulate energy flow through all areas and release all energy blocks or imbalances.

If you detect a possible imbalance in energy, you may be asked what it might mean. It's natural for you to feel completely comfortable and sleepy. You will have a glass of water and a chance to rest and sleep after your diagnosis.

Who could possibly have reflexology?

Everyone can benefit from reflexological treatments from newborn babies to very elderly people. The therapist takes into account your age and health when scheduling the nature and duration of your treatment and adjusts the pressure he or she uses to meet your needs better.

Foot Reflexology Systems in Massage Chairs

Reflexology is a natural method used in a health prevention program. The reflexology of ancient Egypt may trace its origins. Since the Egyptians, a lot has been learned about reflexology. Now, reflexology foot systems with modern technology find their way into massage chairs.

Foot reflexology improves the circulation of the lymph and vascular. It also allows the hormonal system to balance. It is also an effective remedy for diseases of the nervous system. There are many advantages including relaxation when regular foot reflexology massages are provided.

First of all, we must consider certain links between the feet and the rest of the body. Each foot has 7200 endings of the nerves. They offer direct access to the body's circulatory and nervous systems. Another important element is that the feet are the farthest away from the heart, helping to improve circulation.

The theory behind a foot massage in reflexology is based on the principle that reflex points exist. Reflexology uses specific pressures that induce deep relaxation. The nerve endings of the feet are linked to the main bodies of the body.

Massage chairs are made using a mixture of reflexology plates or nodes and an air massage device. A massage chair has specially designed applications to handle various systems for massage reflexology. These technologies bring soothing relief and relaxation.

A reflexology plate is an important development. These specially designed plates are located in the leg rest wells. The feet are placed on top of the plates of reflexology. Such crafted panels activate the trigger points on the feet's soles.

The use of specialized nodes is another strategy. Typically, these nodes are attached to an airbag. The airbag is inflated to activate the reflexological points.

Specially designed airbags are used to provide the side and top of feet for a comfortable massage. The air pressure is used to alleviate and preserve the rigidity of the feet. The airbags either push the feet on or hold them while the specialized nodes push into the trigger points.

The advanced reflexology plates were produced by Panasonic. These can also be removed if the user does not want this kind of massage to be used. Specialized reflexology nodes have been used by other firms such as Sanyo and Omega. Such nodes are attached to airbags that activate the feet's soils.

When these reflexology systems are activated, the reflex points on the bottom of the feet are under pressure. This helps to stimulate numerous nerve endings that help the organ in the body to relax. These systems are very effective and are further improved with every new massage chair generation.

Boost your general well-being by treating foot reflexology. Massage chairs provide the best way to ensure that this type of treatment is available on request. Reflexology causes a deep relaxation called homeostasis. This allows the body to release everyday stress and tension. Use a reflexology massage chair as part of the overall health care program.

You may be surprised for those who consider reflexology simply to be a pleasant foot massage. Reflexology is the gentle manipulation of pressure points towards clear paths for flowing energy. The increased energy then stimulates the body and helps it heal itself.

By comparison to chiropractic and acupuncture reflexology, the individual is supported by a natural process. Different foot areas suspected to be connected to specific glands, organs and limbs are treated to help the body correct itself.

Reflexologists learn about the dynamic reaction mechanism of the body. Based on this experience, they move the feet to activate the reactions in organs and body regions. Reflexology is almost exclusively based on autonomous responses.

What Is the Difference Between Massage and Reflexology?

Simply put, reflexology confines hand and feet to manipulation. Massage therapists work in all parts of the body to relax tight muscles. Massage therapy works to connect the muscles to the nervous system.

Reflexology operates on a believed connection between hands and footpoints to direct energy pathways to the limbs and other parts of the body. Massage acts directly on the muscles and nerves where reflexology induces a tissue reaction at a distance from the point stimulated.

Reflexology aims to improve the functioning of muscles, glands and body systems such as circulatory, digestive and breathing, while massage aims to improve the function of the tissue in the body. Reflexologists only touch hands and feet while massage therapists work throughout the entire body.

What are reflexology advantages?

Reflexologists work on the premise that stress causes Â¾ of all human diseases. Their goal is to reduce stress and to create profound relaxation. Reflexologists learn to reduce discomfort and clear blocked routes to over 14,000 nerves.

Via reflexology, the cardiovascular system can allow blood to flow through the body more efficiently. This also increases the production of vitamins, minerals, and nutrients in the whole body and waste to be extracted. Reflexology helps to balance the whole function of the body.

People who experience reflexology say that they have more time, feel more "centric" and have fewer diseases. We also say that we recover more quickly from illnesses such as cold and flu. Customers who frequently undergo reflexology rely on being more concentrated and alert and on relaxing faster and deeper.

How am I starting?

To start benefiting from reflexology, little is needed. Reflexology is a choice for you regardless of your fitness or health status. You only need a good, authorized reflexologist to book an appointment and try!

Like thousands of others in the Pittsburg area, you too can feel less depressed, happier, healthy and concentrated through reflexology therapy. Most reflexologists provide reduced or complementary therapies for the first time, so you can discover the therapeutic benefits of reflexology for yourself.

Does Foot Reflexology Work?

Reflexology is a massage method that uses direct pressure on the hands and feet. Reflexologists claim that certain points on the feet refer to the specific corpses and areas of the body and that pressure on the points involved affects certain bodies.

Reflexology was developed in the 1930s as a technique by a physical therapist called Eunice Ingham. She consulted with Dr. Riley, a psychiatrist who was an area therapist. He believed that pain could be alleviated and the causes of pain cured by rubbing the ear, tongue, nose and other areas at different points.

The therapist regularly pushes on different points of the feet, generally with his thumbs, during the reflexology session. For reasons I don't understand, we also apply very severe pressure to the extent that it is painful.

Each therapist and client seems to think that reflexology is meant to hurt. Perhaps part of the attraction is that it feels good when they end. I don't know. I don't ask. I don't ask. I don't know.

The truth, of course, is that the body does not reveal the hands or feet. There is no proof that any particular organ dysfunction can be triggered by pressing any particular point on foot.

Why do massage therapists keep believing this and marketing it to their clients? I have no idea. I have no idea. I have no idea. I have no idea. It obviously sounds so silly, especially today, but people are convinced of all sorts of odd ideas.

When reflexology works, with the pressure on your foot, you should be able to improve your gall bladder. You don't have other places to "treat." However, the most obvious fault is that no control group can be compared with. For half an hour, several people sleep and rub their feet to make it a relaxing and soothing experience.

There would be no pressure on certain stages. A general foot massage, unspecified, could be equally soothing and effective. About half an hour, it might be just as nice to lie down and relax or massage some part of your body. It does not mean the curative advantage of reflection itself. This does not, however, preclude reflexologists from claiming the value of therapeutic treatment.

Modern Reflexology

Modern reflexology began in the early 1900s. Dr's led. William H. Fitzgerald, George Starr White and Edwin F. Bowers. They developed "zone therapy," in which they thought the body was "mapped" in various areas. Such areas corresponded to various body structures. Dr. Eunice Ingham is known as the "Mother of Modern Reflexology." By mapping her feet, she expanded on zone treatment.

She found very specific points in the feet and hands relating to the different organs, glands, and structures of the human body, namely: the spinal column. The corresponding organ or gland is activated by activating these points with applied pressure.

How reflexology works should continue your reflexology with a gentle "heating" of the feet. Once complete, the reflexologist starts to exert pressure on certain points on your feet. This is done to activate the pressure point's nerve ending. The corresponding organ or gland is activated in response.

A "crystal deposit" is sometimes found on a particular point. It is assumed that these crystals block the end of the nerve. The reflexologist breaks down these tanks with pressure and relaxation. It opens the pathway between the end of the nerve and the corresponding organ.

Everyone differs in the way their bodies respond to reflexology. Most people will quickly see and hear the impact. Others will need multiple sessions to begin to notice the results they want.

Like all forms of treatment, it depends on the time and severity of the condition. Reflexology is a comprehensive approach and a good choice for certain treatments. The assumption that reflexology works are another secret to positive results. The relation between mind and body is powerful; if you have a positive mental attitude, your body reacts positively.

Here are some of the findings that my clients reported to me: most people reported constipation relief within 3-24 hours.

Menstrual cramp relief.

Stress relief, reflexology is very calming.

Better and longer sleeping at night.

Back pain relief.

Migraine pain relief.

Reflexology is a holistic approach to the care of the body, as is the value of massage therapy. The function of the liver, intestines, skin, circulation and lungs is improved by reflexology. It improves bladder and bowel function.

Reflexology helps to relieve pain through the release of endorphins (the body's natural pain killer). It can help to reduce stress and tiredness. This gives cold relief until you are in a feverish condition. It can help to promote work in premature pregnancies. The unpleasant side effects of various cancer treatments can be supported by reflexology.

Hand Reflexology - A Healing Art

The pressure is a technique that most people know as reflexology to apply to different pressures. Our body is divided into regions, which correspond to the pressure points. The technique can be used on the hands as well as the feet. Hand reflexology dates back to ancient Egypt.

The benefits of hand reflexology are even greater today. Game consoles, computers and other gadgets we use every day make our hands commonly used. Hand reflexology is useful not only for hands overworked but also for the rest of the body.

If you are looking for a way to disrupt tension cycles in your body, hand reflexology needs to be applied. The relevant parts of the body are relaxed by hand, reflexology relaxing pressure sensors.

The relaxation extends across the entire body as the nervous system works. Healing can start, and wellbeing can improve when the body is tired and comfortable. Medical studies have found that reflexology and meditation have a positive effect on the brain and the heart.

Many people are not as conscious of hand reflexology as foot reflexology, but both processes work in the same way. Since the hands are more open, and we work with our hands, many people can work with them better.

Everybody can learn the art of reflexology by hand. It is a simple process of disrupting the stress patterns formed by mixing motion, pressure, and stretches. When you perform reflexology in your hands, make sure that your hands are not overworked. You can wait for a few days for your hands if you feel any pain or discomfort after reflexology.

You can even learn the principles of hand reflexology and use them for yourself. If you need to calm down or feel stressed for a few moments, these strategies are perfect. It is a simple process to identify and know techniques.

A credible source of information. Most services provide step-by-step therapies and maps showing which parts of your hands match areas of your body.

Most people like to use massage equipment to put pressure on. There are wooden devices that can be rolled between your hands to raise successful pressure points. A UK reflexologist, Kevin Kunz, claims that his favorite hand reflexology device is a gold coin. "Grap hands and hold a golf ball between your hands and roll the ball under the thumb through your palm," he suggests.

Reflexology can help the bodies repair themselves; it can be an efficient contact therapy tool as it breaks down stress cycles and relaxes the body. Touch makes a person feel well looked after, creates and binds all people with tactile senses.

There is skepticism about reflexology, but these people do not have to accept that reflexology would benefit from the procedure. We can improve our overall health by stopping a few minutes and doing hand reflexology to relieve the stress patterns which plague us daily.

Foot Reflexology

If your last nerve has "fetus" pain, foot reflexology helps not only soothe and relax your soils and your fur but also restores your body balance. As an ancient healing practice, foot reflexology is based on the theory that feet match all body systems.

Specific pressure is applied in foot reflexology to "reflexes" that result in stress reduction by thumb, finger and hand methods. Foot reflexology also benefits from stress and anxiety relief and overall well-being feelings.

Foot Reflexology maintains the natural balance and is meant to revitalize patients but not as a curing agent. This holistic healing technique is currently useful in determining high stress or stress areas of the body. Since many conditions of health are linked with stress, foot reflexology could prove promising complementary therapy in the modern age.

Both individuals and certified massage therapists find foot reflexology courses not only useful for personal use but also help to enhance trained massage practices. The course in foot-reflexology typically lasts for more than 60 hours but can be completed in a few weeks or in more detail.

Different soccer reflexology programs are offered to the public in detailed workshops and seminars and in continuing education and elective courses in massage schools.

In this particular discipline, there are a growing number of reflexological schools that strictly train and obtain a certificate or diploma. Reflexology research generally involves body and behavioral experiments, stress reduction techniques, how foot (or hands, ears) and reflective structures can be mapped.

Let professional education start in -industries such as massage therapy, cosmetology, acupuncture, oriental medicine, Reiki and more, if you (or anyone that you know) are interested in learning soccer reflexology. In your area, consider vocational school services.

Chinese Reflexology Therapy

Chinese reflexology is a global favorite for advocates of alternative therapies and also known as reflexology, although it can also be more generally known as touch therapy or foot massage.

The Chinese found out that the patient would benefit from the corresponding species that were supposed to have been connected to the pressure point by applying pressure or massage stimulation at certain stages.

This was consistent with the Chinese meridian system or energy channels. In western medicine, it has been explained either as a link through a neural network or as a multitude of interconnecting nerves, or it is simply not explained at all.

While there is a lot of debate among non-alternative Western practitioners and personal views about the validity of the ancient Chinese reflexology method. I recently talked to a podiatrist who believed sincerely in the importance of Chinese reflectivity but acknowledged that it was "sheer quackery" that he was taught in the university.

Nevertheless, the world's demand for reflexology is increasing because it is not intrusive, drug-free and holistic, and because of the ever-growing popularity and acceptability of alternative healing approaches among global populations.

Foot reflexology is by far the most common and successful reflexology therapy under service. This is partly because many professionals specialize in foot reflexology as well as the fact that most people find it especially relaxing and often go to a Foot Reflexology session as an alternative to a massage, not just for their therapeutic benefit.

Nevertheless, Chinese reflexology can also be extended to many parts of the body. It is usually used on the feet, hands, and ears but also on most other parts of the body.

The pressure can be applied with static or massaging pressure. This can be done without creams, oil or device, but Chinese reflexology, like many practices, has been mingled with so many other techniques by multi-disciplinary therapists that it is not uncommon to find reflexology therapists who use pressure and lotions to improve treatment.

reflexology programs like Thai Reflexology also use pressure instruments such as wooden instruments.

A popular trend today is to study and frequently handle Chinese reflexology techniques or to practice them on your partner or children. You can consult a specialist to teach you if you are more a perfectionist or a purist, or you can learn from many excellent books or even YouTube.

Chinese reflexology says it unblocks energy pathways, strengthens the immune system, and helps eliminate toxins that return the body to equilibrium and restore energy

The Benefits of Hand Reflexology

Many people are keen to try this type of alternative medicine, but before embarking on their healing and well-being journey, they would like to know the principles of reflexology. There are numerous reflex points on your feet and hands. If these points are touched and massaged with specific techniques, your body will be affected by the coordination of the organ. The frequent use of hand reflexology will help vital organs unblock the energy within themselves and allow natural healing processes to take place.

One of the greatest advantages of hand reflection is that these techniques allow your body to release the negative feelings in it. Reflexology also helps the body release contaminants and toxins which have been developed over the years. It is important to help your body to detoxify from these toxins because it can decrease your health.

Reflexology helps the body keep energy balances through the opening of blocks within the body. Many things in life can cause energy blockages, but in a few reflexology sessions, they can easily be removed. It opens the circulation lines and helps the body to achieve its optimal performance.

There are specific reflex points directly related to your body's main organs. If you feel symptoms of a disease or condition, then the techniques of reflexology relating to your body can actually help overcome the symptoms.

Reflective technology is not a painful process, and it is gentle and easy to perform techniques. Nevertheless, the advantages of reflexology are remarkable, and many people are shocked by the wellbeing and the fact that they frequently use reflexology.

The Difference Between Foot and Hand Reflexology

There are many similarities between foot reflexology and hand reflexology, and this section will examine how they compare and what benefits reflexology can bring.

The energy system in the body uses hand and foot reflexology to enhance healing and well-being. There are specific reflexes in the feet and hands, and these reflexes are directly related to the major organs of the body.

If specific health problems occur, signs can be avoided, and the body can be healed using reflexology. It's crucial that you place the particular areas in your feet and hands that correspond with your problems.

Using reflexology techniques on your hands or feet (depending upon your condition), the energy levels in your body can be balanced. Reflexology helps these energy points become unblocked, which allows the energy to flow freely and in effect, facilitates the body's natural healing processes.

Reflexology is an alternative form of medicine, and some doctors do not agree to help you treat or resolve physical conditions. But there are many people who have experienced life-changing cures through regular use of reflexology.

When you start applying reflexology techniques in your life, make sure you start with an open mind. The body's energy levels are very adaptive and provide a little more healing power than most people realize. With an open mind about reflexology, you can feel all the advantages of reflexology.

Reflexology therapies and their effects Reflexology treatments provide many advantages, but why should we care about reflexology?

Living in the modern world poses many challenges for people, including how to remain healthy and fit. As a culture, we are often overworked, drained, depressed and just don't care about ourselves. Yet solutions are in place to address all these issues.

One such technology is a medicine known as reflexology, which massages certain reflexes or pressure points in the hands, feet, and rocks, referring to various areas of the body. For instance, a reflex in hand may relieve back muscles or alleviate knee discomfort.

Reflexology is a holistic therapy, which means it is normal. More and more, the key to preserving people's health can be found in natural cures and not in the use of toxic medicines.

Reflexology works by stimulating the points of reflection in the hands, feet, and ears. Such areas are connected to all body parts, including muscles, tissues, and organs. The coinciding part of the body is harmonized and cleaned by applying gentle pressure in these areas.

Reflexology treatments work as they relieve stress and encourage a cure of the body by reducing inflammation in the affected areas.

After their first experience with reflexology, most people will probably conclude that they have been to the spa rather than therapy. Typically a visit ends with an interview with a professional reflexologist.

Depending on where the procedure will continue, the patient will be asked to sit or sit. Then the reflexologist kneads his hands and feet and applies gentle pressure on the areas that support the part of the body that needs relief. Patients may need more than one treatment to do everything their body needs.

The benefits of reflexology are numerous. These provide relief from pain and stress, increased blood flow and harmonization, and toxin removal. Further specifics are given on how reflexology addresses some of our most important health challenges. Stress in the body can occur in various ways, most often in tension, headaches, migraines, constipation, and acne.

Reflexology can help relax the stress on the body and alleviate the symptoms. The normal and effective pain relief is another benefit of reflexology. Pain is often a warning sign that when something is wrong, your body sends out.

Too often, pain occurs as a side effect when the body is repaired by medication or operation. Reflexology can contribute to relieving this pain by leading the organ to heal itself by releasing endorphins into the body.

People with problems like asthma, bronchitis, premenstrual syndrome, and other health problems also saw great improvements in the practice of reflexology.

A patient, however, doesn't have to wait until he finds a trained reflexologist. Let your body enjoy the benefits of reflexology, which has proved to be one of the best alternative treatments for the wellbeing of the body.

Chapter 12

Percussion Massage Therapy

Percussion Therapy is associated with different types of massage therapy techniques and is considered to be ideal for different types of clinical practice.

The number of medical percussion massage therapy tools is widely used by professionals and individuals throughout the world for avoiding the risks associated with internal systems, and few common percussion therapies include respiratory therapy.

Valuable ideas were developed to reduce stress, in addition to myofascial release, deep muscle therapy, trigger reduction, lactic acid insert relief, muscle spasm treatment, rehabilitation, muscle pond reduction, and postural drainage.

We should remember that many people are now going for massage therapy, and they have confidence that quality percussion massage therapy can relieve all tension, and serious physical and mental problems appear to be related to their social, personal and business lives.

Scout's honor that massage therapy can genuinely cure your pride and it is no strange that percussion therapy should saturate your body to the highest degree of comfort and convenience and thus encourage you to forget all the chaos and disturbances.

The term "percussion massage therapy" has countless benefits; it informally guarantees that the series of rapid, relaxing, light and striking actions are usually applied with the aid of alternate hands in rapid intervals.

Mostly 2 acts can be seen as the fundamental percussion strokes, specifically as cupping and hacking: these strokes can be performed on different parts of the body, and the systems become more effective, for example in the thigh and upper body areas when both are used on a body with a large muscular / fleshy region. Certain movements devoted to percussion stimulation are pounding, throbbing and rubbing.

The set of these movements often start from the area of your wrist rather than from your shoulders, elbows, and head, yet it is the basic thing that every therapist must be aware of because the majority of the therapist is doing percussion therapy and making movements of the elbows and the shoulders.

Cupping is a sensitive part of the therapy usually done with hands, turning upside down and forming a hollow curvature.

Thus the therapist pushes the cushions at the fast pace as a result of which a vacuum is created which is released when the therapist lifts his or her hands, and the performance sounds hollow, as the care of horses. This art of massage is often known as Cupping sometimes also recognized as clapping. It shows the word "cupped" hands in both terms.

Hacking is a second part of the percussion therapy, which is without a doubt the best-prescribed massage procedure, the same type of treatment that we often see in films, it is done at both sides of the screen, and the practitioner places the hands over the body position, two palms facing one another, and holds the thumbs at the top of their foot.

The last therapist moves up and down the hands in rapid succession in the rhythmic interval. These movements are often made to wake the person up.

The following move is Flicking, much like Hacking, and the word finger hacking is also intended to be represented. In this part of the work, the therapist must flex the wrists slowly by connecting the finger sides to the body without using a hand edge. Flicking is a type of relaxing movement that can make your body's muscles lasting.

The last steps in percussion massage therapy are to beat and pound, the therapist performs these with his hands, and the hands of the massager can be clenched slightly with his fist.

Beating is carried out by means of an undefined boundary with closed fists and punching is carried out on the surface of the body with the two hands. Both movements are managed to achieve better results in quick succession.

Percussion massage treatments are very momentary and can be very effective in relaxing muscles. Blood circulation increases, and blood flows very rapidly into the body. Percussion therapy can boost muscle tone working power and enable muscles to contract and expand with good grace.

CHAPTER 13

Massage Therapy – Preparing the Area

To offer a really good therapeutic massage, a person must spend time training before practicing therapeutic massage for a few more years. Nevertheless, through various simple techniques, a person learns how to give another person a very successful but safe and simple massage that is totally satisfying.

What is crucial is to ensure that the area where you will massage is properly established. Nevertheless, when planning the area where massage therapy is going to take place, four things have to be done very carefully.

1 Surface–The surface on which the person will lie during a massage therapy session is important not only to be comfortable but also to provide support and to be firm.

You can either buy a massage table or use a futon or additional firm mattress on which the individual can lie. Never use any form of furniture that doesn't give the person with the massage enough support as it puts unspeakable pressure on their joints.

2 Room-When you set up your massage area, please don't need a room in your home that you can actually use for a massage. Why not use this for your massage therapy sessions if you have a spare bedroom?

However, you can still use it while guests stay away from your massage therapy facilities. Make sure you also have an extra pillow, which you can use to comfort yourself. Plus, if you can make sure the room is large enough to straddle the person who has the massage therapy easily.

3 Create the right atmosphere-It is important for everyone to relax more easily in the area it takes place when providing massage treatment. So why not light a few bells and make some lights visible in the room and put some very soft and gentle music to listen to while you're working on them. If you have to place the lock on the door so that nobody can work in the room suddenly.

4 Clothing-Some people may be embarrassed because they have to be naked before you. Therefore, recommend that you bring any underwear that is comfortable to wear and that you do not feel bad if a massage oil gets on it by accident.

Even if they like to sit on their bra while you do the massage, then let them do so. Even if you might find it difficult to perform a massage therapy session on a woman who wears a bra, you will soon find ways to overcome this challenge.

It is important that you keep in mind that the individual finds a way to relax while preparing the area for the massage therapy session. So by holding this in mind, you should be able to easily accomplish this.

CHAPTER 14

ARE THERE RISKS INVOLVED IN MASSAGE THERAPY?

Regardless of how it was phrased, one question a prospective massage therapist must always pose is, "Which health conditions would you find to be preventative of massage therapy and why?"

Whether in such terms or in other phrases, is the correct answer? "There are certain conditions of health which have to be omitted from massage therapy.

Massage therapy takes various forms, impacting the body differently.

There are also many different types of cancers and patients may receive different therapies at various stages. In some cases and in certain forms of massage therapy, the results can be life-threatening while in other cases, the results can be extraordinarily useful.

Due to this nature, it is important to consult the physician who knows the specifics of the case involved before continuing with any form of massage therapy.

The potential risks involved in massage treatment of cancer patients do not generally outweigh the principle of massage therapy as a whole, but this does mean extra caution and, possibly, mild to severe modification.

And the health hazards are as follows: bone fractures. Many forms of cancer and therapies weaken the bones so that they can crack under strain quickly.

Bleeding

Many patients with cancer tend to bleed easily. Massage of deep tissue can cause hazardous internal bleeding.

Dissemination of cancer tumors.

The effects of massage therapy on tumors are under continuous debate. Some say that applying strong pressure in the area where the tumor is present causes metastasis (breakdown and spreading or increasing its growth rate). Others, however, reject that claim as unfounded and false. It is best to play safely and not massage the tumor area or the soft tissue that surrounds it.

Lymphedema (the deposition of lymph in the soft tissue contributing to limb swelling).

Some forms of massage therapy that contribute to lymphedema in patients whose lymph nodes have been damaged by cancer.

Symptoms close to flu.

Chemotherapy patients may often develop symptoms that look and feel like flu after certain forms of massage therapy have been administered.

Cancer patients often have a lot of pain and most massage treatments can provide some temporary pain after treatment. This can turn into additional pain when too much of it is present and practically intolerable.

Post-operative surgery.

Soon after surgery, both on the outside and internally, the wound is still physically healed. Pressure can cause a number of risky health problems, such as reopening of the incision, internal and/or external bleeding or clotting of the blood, etc.

Conditions of skin.

Areas where the skin is irritated, inflamed, or affected by rashes or sores should not be massaged as the condition can worsen.

Even if all the risks listed above are taken into account, massage therapy can still be very effective for most people in most cases. Rather than dismiss it entirely because of specific concerns, I would encourage a doctor to consult.

CHAPTER 15

Understand What to Expect During Massage Therapy

Massage therapy is discreet and in private so that a customer feels secure. It has been around for a very long time, so there are many various variations. A massage receiver decides which form of massage he or she will get.

During recovery, other tools and materials are used. Physical therapists can use massage to support patients in their recovery. The treatment is guaranteed to be fun and relaxing because you know what to expect during the therapy.

Before the first treatment, the therapist will ask questions about a customer's health and history. The therapist may also inquire if there is any discomfort and if the client is under stress. In answering these questions honestly, the therapist can ensure that a customer receives a massage safely.

The actual massage takes place in a private room. After a customer arrives in a room, they have the option of unloading but only to their comfort. They are then put under a sheet or blanket on the table. The doctor will only show the part of the body massaged.

Massage theory and technique date from the earliest times. There are many styles produced around the globe by different cultures. Whatever form of massage the same results are obtained.

Many impressive findings include increased breathing, relief of pain and good old relaxation. Swedish massage is a very frequent type of massage. Swedish is characterized by long, flowing, light strokes often facing the center.

Stone therapy is another well-known massage. The therapist uses warm or cold rocks to put on certain parts of the body of a person. They can also be held in the hands of the therapist for a massage. The stones are usually flat and even river blocks.

A massage is usually given in a professional setting on a bed. The table can be portable or stationary, depending on whether a massage is offered in the therapist's office or in another location. New linens are going to be on the bed. We help to ensure security and privacy for a consumer.

A massage therapist uses his hands, backstabbers or a massage mix. Typically hypoallergenic lotions, oils or creams are used to minimize skin pressure during the massage.

So make relaxing easier, the room is warm and comfortable. The lighting is often dim and candles can be lit. Music can be played in the background softly. Lightly fragrant oils, called aromatherapy, are sometimes used to add to the room's ambiance.

Doctors can suggest that a patient receive a physical therapist massage. Physical therapists can use massage to help a patient recover more easily. The same tools and equipment a physical therapist use as a massage therapist.

Massage is almost safe for anyone. It's done in private. There are many different massage styles, and there's something for everyone. As part of physical therapy or as prescribed by a doctor, a patient can receive massage.

Since there are so many different kinds of massage, something for everyone will surely be there. A client can relax and make the most of a session by knowing what to expect during massage treatment.

In the past, a torn muscle could finish a career for athletes. Athletes today enjoy specialized massage therapy that extends their careers. Massage therapy equipment with massage tables pliable into suitcase size has become quite sophisticated.

Chapter 16

What Is the Best Type of Massage Therapy for Me?

Massage therapy is the broad term used to describe the various techniques of manual (hands-to-hand) therapy that is used to promote tissue health. The type of massage therapy a person receives depends heavily on his or her particular problem or disability and health. There is something for all and consumers need to test their options and find out what works for them.

The most popular type of massage is the Swedish massage, which Per Henrik Ling developed in the early 1800s and late 1700s. The Swedish massage techniques are long smooth strokes (effleurage), kneading of tissue (petrissage), tapping and can be used to relax or increase muscle tone depending on application and technique.

Pressure can be very light or deep, depending on your therapist, needs and pressure tolerance. Certain techniques that may require further or advanced training can be used during massage therapy, consisting primarily of Swedish technology.

All components of Swedish techniques are addressed in relaxation, exercise, maternity, child and geriatric massage.

Relaxation massage appears to be slower and rhythmic than a therapeutic massage and its primary objective is to improve consumer relaxation.

In child, massage therapists teach parents how to work with their own children, a great bonding experience that parents can help relieve colic and help their children to sleep better. With specific groups or disorders, such as breastfeeding or geriatric massage, procedures should be adapted to suit the customer's needs.

Sports massage therapy involves not only Scandinavian methods but also relaxation techniques, which include "strong inhibition." The pre-event sports massage therapy uses rhythmic movements to warm up and stretch muscles, preparing them for demand. Sports therapy after the event is more gradual and performed to relieve pain, swelling, help to remove metabolic waste and reduce recovery time. Massage therapies for athletes and fitness enthusiasts are also a great maintenance tool that offers the ability to address and optimize muscle imbalances and injuries.

Deep tissue massage therapy consists mainly of Swedish procedures used at a lower level of the tissue. In order to effectively perform all massages, but especially deep tissue, muscles must be warmed up superficially to allow the therapist to penetrate the deeper layers and to tackle constraints.

The use of a hi-lo table and specialized training is suitable for therapists who want to practice "deep tissue" to help them maintain their own body, backs and joint health. To new massage therapy clients, it is best to treat deep tissue as it is not appropriate for everybody and can be uncomfortable for someone not used to manual therapy.

Myofascial trigger point therapy is also known as the release of trigger points. A myofascial trigger is a region that can be hyper irritated in a tight muscle band. The purpose of this procedure is to reduce or eliminate the trigger point and so alleviate pain.

Reference pain often has a very specific pattern depending on the muscle it is located and can often occur in an apparently unrelated location. Trigger point therapy is incorporated into Swedish massage treatments which help to warm and stretch tissue before and after release.

Friction or friction therapy is a very precise, localized technique used to break down adhesion and scar tissue that can cause discomfort and hinder movement. Friction therapy is not used alone, but it is integrated into a routine where Swedish techniques are used to heat tissue and to help circulation to remove post-friction metabolic waste.

Myofascial release procedure, also known as the fascial release, consists of the stimulation and stretching of the body's fascial-connective tissue that encloses muscles, nerves, organs and bones. To effectively stabilize and secure the tissues no oil or other medium is used, as in most myofascial procedures, "gliding" over tissue is ineffective.

Manual lymphatic drainage is a sequence of gentle motions used to promote lymphatic fluid flow in the body, thus relieving pain and inflammation, also known as lymphatic, lymph and lymphatic massage.

This kind of treatment is ideal for helping to reduce swelling after an injury and also for reducing swelling following surgery. MLD, as is widely known, is also used with great success for women with mastectomy, but special training is needed when lymph nodes are removed for therapists to treat.

The main focus of most of the massage therapy instruction is on Swedish techniques, but the above modalities can be practiced either as an addendum or as a supplement to the Swedish massage.

The active release is a proprietary procedure that involves different movements during stimulation of the tissue. The term "active," refers to the fact that the patient contracts his / her muscles voluntarily in the form of techniques. Specialized training and certification are required for this therapy.

CHAPTER 17

When Should You Get Massage Therapy?

When should you undergo bodywork or massage therapy?

The question arises even more than you might think. People ask if they should obtain morning, midday or evening massage therapy.

You would like to ask if you should relax before starting to hurt or wait until the muscle pain becomes intolerable. Many people ask if it's easier before, during or after sports.

I respond to all of these questions during my San Antonio massage Therapy and Bodywork clinic, Massage By Ben, by saying, "You will come every day." Obviously, my reaction is language-in-cheek.

I clarify then that it's good but unnecessary to get massage therapy every day and maybe cost-prohibitive. In addition, when and how often you undergo massage therapy is dependent on the objectives you want to follow with massage therapy. How we reach your goals with massage therapy is more important than just a simple question and answer in this chapter.

This should be a living conversation between you and your bodyworker or massage therapist, but what about the fundamental issues? Let's respond to those: Q1. Should I have my morning, midday or evening massage therapy? I don't want to sleep at night, but during the day I want to feel better.

A1. Most people worry about this one, but you shouldn't think about that. Massage therapy relaxes, and some people sleep during the session, but you will not be tired afterward.

Most people actually feel more calm and comfortable after their massage therapy. Still, no matter at what time you get your massage, when you finally go to bed, you will probably sleep better. So if it's easy for you, take your massage therapy.

Q2. Should I undergo my massage therapy before my muscle pain starts, or should I wait for it to hurt before I seek massage treatment?

A2. It is much easier in my experience to get massage therapy to prevent muscle pain or muscle pain from returning. Many massage therapists and clients claim that waiting for moderate pain makes it easier for them to find a source, but that rarely happens. Get help early. Get help.

Q3. Will I receive massage therapy before, during, or after sports?

A3. Yes. There are advanced massage services to support you in your health and athletic activities. Sports Massages are often categorized into pre-event, inter-event and post-event techniques to improve performance and assist in rehabilitation. If in each step of your operation, you do not have access to massage therapy, choose what is most important to you–success or recovery.

I still think if you can come in every day because a "massage a day" is perfect, then it really is a "massage a day." For course, even if you undergo massage therapy and bodywork once, the benefits are open to you.

CHAPTER 18

MOBILE MASSAGE THERAPY

Accumulation of everyday stress Long hours work on your computer can result in stress, muscle stress, injury or pain that can drain your body, mind or emotion. This can negatively affect your social life as well as your work.

Since stress reduction is the most important benefit of massage therapy, overall health can be improved and adverse effects of stress minimized or prevented. It can reduce pain continuously, prevent injury and maintain health. It is an essential part of physically and mentally healthy living because it relieves stress, which accounts for 90% of illness and pain.

The massage affects the inner organs and regions isolated from the therapeutic area by the autonomous nervous system due to the reflex effects. This encourages relaxation, reduces pain, improves mood and clarity of mind.

Massage can be used to relax or have fun and to recover from surgery, injury or poor health. It enhances blood and lymph supply, increases the natural killer cells and lymphocytes that destroy cancer cells;

Improves mood through the increase of serotonin and dopamine, and alleviates pain through the increased use of endorphins in pain control.

Transforms and rejuvenates, restores equilibrium to your body and life, so you can take it all your way. Digestion, joint mobility, muscle relaxation, spasm, and cramp relief can be facilitated.

Massage therapy is more sophisticated and effective when it moves into new spaces, such as the fastest expanding massage method.

Bodywork as a medical therapy

The instruction in massage therapy was an important part of medical massage and nursing until the mid-1950s, when the rapid development and almost exclusive use of technology during the twentieth hundred nearly dropped to nothing.

Manual therapy was no longer considered appropriate in regular hospital care. It is now clear; however, that massage in the hospital is necessary to give a sense of completeness and lack of care because of an increasing focus on the specialization in the increasing heterogeneity of hospitalization.

Medical massage uses traditional massage movements, which are then changed to treat, for example, cancer patients, hospitals and pregnant women. The therapist can go to a hospital, an ambulatory clinic or a mobile therapy to provide a personalized treatment protocol for the patient.

The doctor pays close attention to the side-effects of curative therapy in the massage care of the cancer patient to assess an appropriate technique. In this situation, the treatment focuses on certain side effects such as pain, lymphedema, scariness, nausea, stress, sleeplessness, exhaustion, frustration, depression, anxiety.

Cancer massage is, therefore, a special treatment that complements curative medical treatments such as procedure, chemotherapy and radiation.

Therefore, more knowledge of medical procedures, pathologies and side effects than ordinary therapy is needed. If not known, the patient is affected, because the therapist cannot alter the procedure or create a qualified treatment protocol.

The practitioner will also take into consideration musculoskeletal problems caused by the weight of the fetus that affects the center of gravity of the body during pregnancy massage.

In this case, the main focus of care is upper and lower back pain, sacroiliac and lower abdominal pain. The therapist should also be alert to acute medical conditions like deep vein thrombosis and preeclampsia, both of which may be fatal if not medically treated.

Massage reduces pain and stress is the biggest advantage. Bodywork has a broad application in the clinic. Because stress causes a wide range of physical and psychological problems, the massage may help alleviate these symptoms.

Massage relief is a major benefit and tension that helps to alleviate muscle strain, facilitates relaxation and avoids lower back, neck and shoulder pain, breastfeeding, bedsores, serious burns, iliotibial band disease and damage to the spinal cord, as well as systemic change including cystic fibrosis, ADDs, fibromyalgia, asthma, autism, diabetes.

Sleep disorders, exhaustion from cancer, diabetes, high blood pressure, spinal cord injuries, reduced immune systems, post-operative surgery, autism, eating disorders, age-related disorders and cessation of smoking may be massages.

Bodywork, like shiatsu and acupuncture, offers a non-medical, non-invasive approach that bases people on the natural capacity of the body to heal itself.

Pregnancy bodywork

Huge physical, mental and emotional changes affect the lifestyle, career and family and friends relationship. Massage helps you implement these enhancements effectively. Massage treatment increases overall health, reduces stress, and alleviates muscle discomfort and pain in pregnancy. It explains many skeletal, muscular and circulatory problems caused by the hormone changes during pregnancy.

Massage relieves lower back, hip and leg pain, edema, diarrhea, heartburn, and constipation. Regular massage lowers anxiety and reduces stress hormones. Job is easier and simpler because children are safer. There are fewer obstacles, such as low birth weight and premature birth.

CONCLUSION

Massage therapy is better used as most other medical techniques to prevent injury to your body. Too many people remain there until a real injury occurs before they are searching for massage therapy as a viable option.

In research, I find stress and neck pain the most common problems as a result of inadequate posture at a desk, tendonitis in the hands, and lower back and sciatic nerve pain. All of these issues can be avoided if your weekly schedule involves daily massages.

Injury is most commonly reported in muscle groups that don't get regular workouts every week, so discomfort is not uncommon while sitting at a desk for 6 to 9 hours a day. Problematic muscle areas will become compressed and may cause problems, sciatic damage, and tendonitis.

It is necessary to encourage patients to take short breaks if they can, walk before or after lunch or try to stretch their muscles in a meeting room. Consistent massages can also help and I recommend a massage every two weeks, depending on the discomfort.

The overall objective of massage therapy is to relieve pain and stress. Depending on the amount of pain felt, different techniques and criteria are used.

Massage therapy not only offers the means to reduce pain but also provides you with some time alone. I figure out that some of my clients use massage therapy both for medical purposes and for the chance to relax and to settle for a while.

People who come for daily massage therapy usually sleep well, and when the human body relax, it will heal faster. The value of massage therapy is immense. Most of my clients cannot believe how well they feel after a 1-hour session the very next day.

Even children of all ages are greatly benefited by massages. With children I typically want to start with a 30-minute block of time, depending on the size. It is great for hyperactivity, discomfort, insomnia and helps with increasing pain.

Mothers and fathers in some hospitals can be trained for simple massage techniques to treat their own children at home. This is an incredible way for them to communicate with their children through the power of touch.

I usually recommend that you start with a 60-minute time block to see how your body responds and tweak the massage. Many people can be responsive to certain massage techniques and can only take 1/2 hour, while some people are most likely to benefit from 90 minutes.

Everyone is different and every therapy session should be tailored to the specific needs of that client. Different types of massage therapy can also be used according to the state of the client: treatment with hot stones, maternity massages, and sports massages.

A therapeutic massage can be given to people of any age, as long as it is provided by a qualified therapist. I advise all clients to consider whether they have reimbursement programs for this kind of therapy and whether they want to make sure they accept it and use it.

www.ingramcontent.com/pod-product-compliance
Lightning Source LLC
Chambersburg PA
CBHW071415210526
45465CB00001B/394